EARLY DEVELOPMENT OF TOTAL HIP REPLACEMENT

The transcript of a Witness Seminar held by the Wellcome Trust Centre for the History of Medicine at UCL, London, on 14 March 2006

Edited by L A Reynolds and E M Tansey

Volume 29   2006

First published by the Wellcome Trust Centre
for the History of Medicine at UCL, 2007

The Wellcome Trust Centre for the History of Medicine
at UCL is funded by the Wellcome Trust, which is
a registered charity, no. 210183.

ISBN 978 085484 111 0

All volumes are freely available online following the links to Publications/Wellcome Witnesses at
www.ucl.ac.uk/histmed

CONTENTS

ILLUSTRATIONS AND CREDITS

Appendix 3: Selected prosthetic hips

Abbreviations

BOA	British Orthopaedic Association
BOSG	British Orthopaedic Study Group
BSI	British Standards Institution
CEN	Comité Européen de Normalisation, the European Committee for Standardization, Brussels, Belgium at www.cenorm.be
DoH	Department of Health
FDA	US Food and Drug Administration
HAC	hydroxyapatite coating
HDP	high-density polyethylene
ISO	Interational Organization for Standardization, Genève, Switzerland at www.iso.org/isoenCatalogueListPage.CatalogueList
LFA	low-friction arthroplasty
MCA	Medicines Control Agency
MDA	Medical Devices Agency
MHRA	Medicines and Healthcare Products Regulatory Agency
MRC	Medical Research Council
NHS	National Health Service
NICE	National Institute for Clinical Excellence
NJR	National Joint Registry for England and Wales
PMMA	polymethylmethacrylate
PTFE	polytetrafluoroethylene
RNOH	Royal National Orthopaedic Hospital, Stanmore, Middlesex at www.rnoh.nhs.uk/about_the_RNOH/

THA   total hip arthroplasty

THR   total hip replacement

UHMWPE ultra-high molecular weight polyethylene

UMIST   University of Manchester Institute of Technology, which merged with the Victoria University of Manchester to become the University of Manchester in 2004.

WITNESS SEMINARS:
MEETINGS AND PUBLICATIONS [1]

In 1990 the Wellcome Trust created a History of Twentieth Century Medicine Group, associated with the Academic Unit of the Wellcome Institute for the History of Medicine, to bring together clinicians, scientists, historians and others interested in contemporary medical history. Among a number of other initiatives the format of Witness Seminars, used by the Institute of Contemporary British History to address issues of recent political history, was adopted, to promote interaction between these different groups, to emphasize the potential benefits of working jointly, and to encourage the creation and deposit of archival sources for present and future use. In June 1999 the Governors of the Wellcome Trust decided that it would be appropriate for the Academic Unit to enjoy a more formal academic affiliation and turned the Unit into the Wellcome Trust Centre for the History of Medicine at UCL from 1 October 2000. The Wellcome Trust continues to fund the Witness Seminar programme via its support for the Centre.

The Witness Seminar is a particularly specialized form of oral history, where several people associated with a particular set of circumstances or events are invited to come together to discuss, debate, and agree or disagree about their memories. To date, the History of Twentieth Century Medicine Group has held 45 such meetings, most of which have been published, as listed on pages xv–xxiii.

Subjects are usually proposed by, or through, members of the Programme Committee of the Group, which includes professional historians of medicine, practicing scientists and clinicians, and once an appropriate topic has been agreed, suitable participants are identified and invited. This inevitably leads to further contacts, and more suggestions of people to invite. As the organization of the meeting progresses, a flexible outline plan for the meeting is devised, usually with assistance from the meeting's chairman, and some participants are invited to 'set the ball rolling' on particular themes, by speaking for a short period to initiate and stimulate further discussion.

---

[1] The following text also appears in the 'Introduction' to recent volumes of Wellcome Witnesses to Twentieth Century Medicine published by the Wellcome Trust and the Wellcome Trust Centre for the History of Medicine at UCL.

Each meeting is fully recorded, the tapes are transcribed and the unedited transcript is immediately sent to every participant. Each is asked to check his or her own contributions and to provide brief biographical details. The editors turn the transcript into readable text, and participants' minor corrections and comments are incorporated into that text, while biographical and bibliographical details are added as footnotes, as are more substantial comments and additional material provided by participants. The final scripts are then sent to every contributor, accompanied by forms assigning copyright to the Wellcome Trust. Copies of all additional correspondence received during the editorial process are deposited with the records of each meeting in Archives and Manuscripts, Wellcome Library, London.

As with all our meetings, we hope that even if the precise details of some of the technical sections are not clear to the non-specialist, the sense and significance of the events will be understandable. Our aim is for the volumes that emerge from these meetings to inform those with a general interest in the history of modern medicine and medical science; to provide historians with new insights, fresh material for study, and further themes for research; and to emphasize to the participants that events of the recent past, of their own working lives, are of proper and necessary concern to historians.

[†]Died 13 December 2006

ACKNOWLEDGEMENTS

'Total hip replacement' was suggested as a suitable topic for a Witness Seminar by Dr Francis Neary and Mr Krishna (Ravi) Kunzru, who assisted us in planning the meeting. We are very grateful to them for their input and to Mr Alan Lettin for his excellent chairing of the occasion. We are particularly grateful to Dr Francis Neary and Professor John Pickstone for writing such a useful Introduction to these published proceedings, and to Professor Christopher Colton and Dr Carole Reeves, who read through earlier drafts of the transcript, and offered helpful comments and advice. Our additional thanks go to Professor Alan Swanson, Mr Victor Wheble and Mr Jeffrey Hallett, President of the ISO/TC150 Committee, for their help preparing the appendices for publication. We consulted those involved with the early development of the Charnley, Exeter, ICLH, McKee, McMinn, Ring and Stanmore prostheses who approved the details in Appendix 3 and suggested other changes. We thank the contributors and Professor Colton for their help with the Glossary; and Mr Paul Beverley, Archive Publications, Norwich; Professor Michael Wroblewski, Mr Paul Siney and Ms Patricia Fleming, John Charnley Research Institute, Wrightington Hospital; Mr John Timperley, Exeter Hip Centre; Professor John Paul; Dr Paul Unwin, Stanmore Implants Worldwide Ltd, Centre for Biomedical Engineering (UCL); Mr Chris Carter, Wellcome Trust Medical Photo Library, London; and Mr Bhavik Samani, acting manager, Computer Learning Centre, Whipps Cross Medical Education Centre for their assistance. For permission to reproduce the images included here, we thank Lady Charnley, the John Charnley Trust, Mr Harry Craven, Mr Joseph Daniel of the McMinn Centre, Ms Clare Darrah, the *Eastern Evening News,* Professor Michael Freeman, Mrs Phyllis Hampson, Mr Kevin Hardinge, Howorth Airtech Ltd, the *Journal of Bone and Joint Surgery,* Mr John Kirkup, Mr Ravi Kunzru, Mr Alan Lettin, Professor Robin Ling, Dr Francis Neary, Mr John Read, Mr Peter Ring, Sir Rodney Sweetnam, the Wellcome Photo Library, Mr Victor Wheble and Mr Michael Wilson.

As with all our meetings, we depend a great deal on our colleagues at the Wellcome Trust to ensure their smooth running: the Audiovisual Department, the Medical Photographic Library and the Wellcome Library; Mr Akio Morishima, who has supervised the design and production of this volume; our indexer, Ms Liza Furnival; and our readers, Ms Fiona Plowman and Mr Simon

Reynolds. Mrs Jaqui Carter is our transcriber, and Mrs Wendy Kutner and Dr Daphne Christie assist us in running the meetings. Finally we thank the Wellcome Trust for supporting this programme.

Tilli Tansey

Lois Reynolds

Wellcome Trust Centre for the History of Medicine at UCL

HISTORY OF TWENTIETH CENTURY MEDICINE WITNESS SEMINARS, 1993–2007

1993   **Monoclonal antibodies**

1994   **The early history of renal transplantation**

        Pneumoconiosis of coal workers

1995   **Self and non-self: A history of autoimmunity**

        Ashes to ashes: The history of smoking and health

        Oral contraceptives

        Endogenous opiates

1996   **Committee on Safety of Drugs**

        Making the body more transparent: The impact of nuclear magnetic resonance and magnetic resonance imaging

1997   **Research in general practice**

        Drugs in psychiatric practice

        The MRC Common Cold Unit

        The first heart transplant in the UK

1998   **Haemophilia: Recent history of clinical management**

        Obstetric ultrasound: Historical perspectives

        Post penicillin antibiotics

        Clinical research in Britain, 1950–1980

PUBLISHED MEETINGS

'…Few books are so intellectually stimulating or uplifting'.
Journal of the Royal Society of Medicine (1999) **92:** 206–8,
review of vols 1 and 2

'…This is oral history at its best…all the volumes make compulsive reading…they are, primarily, important historical records'.
British Medical Journal (2002) **325:** 1119, review of the series

Technology transfer in Britain: The case of monoclonal antibodies
Self and non-self: A history of autoimmunity
Endogenous opiates
The Committee on Safety of Drugs
In: Tansey E M, Catterall P P, Christie D A, Willhoft S V, Reynolds L A. (eds) (1997) *Wellcome Witnesses to Twentieth Century Medicine.* Volume 1. London: The Wellcome Trust, 135pp. ISBN 1 869835 79 4

Making the human body transparent: The impact of NMR and MRI
Research in general practice
Drugs in psychiatric practice
The MRC Common Cold Unit
In: Tansey E M, Christie D A, Reynolds L A. (eds) (1998) *Wellcome Witnesses to Twentieth Century Medicine.* Volume 2. London: The Wellcome Trust, 282pp. ISBN 1 869835 39 5

Early heart transplant surgery in the UK
In: Tansey E M, Reynolds L A. (eds) (1999) *Wellcome Witnesses to Twentieth Century Medicine.* Volume 3. London: The Wellcome Trust, 72pp. ISBN 1 841290 07 6

Haemophilia: Recent history of clinical management
In: Tansey E M, Christie D A. (eds) (1999) *Wellcome Witnesses to Twentieth Century Medicine.* Volume 4. London: The Wellcome Trust, 90pp. ISBN 1 841290 08 4

Looking at the unborn: Historical aspects of obstetric ultrasound
In: Tansey E M, Christie D A. (eds) (2000) *Wellcome Witnesses to Twentieth Century Medicine.* Volume 5. London: The Wellcome Trust, 80pp. ISBN 1 841290 11 4

Post penicillin antibiotics: From acceptance to resistance?
In: Tansey E M, Reynolds L A. (eds) (2000) *Wellcome Witnesses to Twentieth Century Medicine*. Volume 6. London: The Wellcome Trust, 71pp.
ISBN 1 841290 12 2

Clinical research in Britain, 1950–1980
In: Reynolds L A, Tansey E M. (eds) (2000) *Wellcome Witnesses to Twentieth Century Medicine*. Volume 7. London: The Wellcome Trust, 74pp.
ISBN 1 841290 16 5

Intestinal absorption
In: Christie D A, Tansey E M. (eds) (2000) *Wellcome Witnesses to Twentieth Century Medicine*. Volume 8. London: The Wellcome Trust, 81pp.
ISBN 1 841290 17 3

Neonatal intensive care
In: Christie D A, Tansey E M. (eds) (2001) *Wellcome Witnesses to Twentieth Century Medicine*. Volume 9. London: The Wellcome Trust Centre for the History of Medicine at UCL, 84pp. ISBN 0 854840 76 1

British contributions to medical research and education in Africa after the Second World War
In: Reynolds L A, Tansey E M. (eds) (2001) *Wellcome Witnesses to Twentieth Century Medicine*. Volume 10. London: The Wellcome Trust Centre for the History of Medicine at UCL, 93pp. ISBN 0 854840 77 X

Childhood asthma and beyond
In: Reynolds L A, Tansey E M. (eds) (2001) *Wellcome Witnesses to Twentieth Century Medicine*. Volume 11. London: The Wellcome Trust Centre for the History of Medicine at UCL, 74pp. ISBN 0 854840 78 8

Maternal care
In: Christie D A, Tansey E M. (eds) (2001) *Wellcome Witnesses to Twentieth Century Medicine*. Volume 12. London: The Wellcome Trust Centre for the History of Medicine at UCL, 88pp. ISBN 0 854840 79 6

Population-based research in south Wales: The MRC Pneumoconiosis Research Unit and the MRC Epidemiology Unit
In: Ness A R, Reynolds L A, Tansey E M. (eds) (2002) *Wellcome Witnesses to Twentieth Century Medicine*. Volume 13. London: The Wellcome Trust Centre for the History of Medicine at UCL, 74pp. ISBN 0 854840 81 8

Peptic ulcer: Rise and fall
In: Christie D A, Tansey E M. (eds) (2002) *Wellcome Witnesses to Twentieth Century Medicine*. Volume 14. London: The Wellcome Trust Centre for the History of Medicine at UCL, 143pp. ISBN 0 854840 84 2

Leukaemia
In: Christie D A, Tansey E M. (eds) (2003) *Wellcome Witnesses to Twentieth Century Medicine*. Volume 15. London: The Wellcome Trust Centre for the History of Medicine at UCL, 86pp. ISBN 0 85484 087 7

The MRC Applied Psychology Unit
In: Reynolds L A, Tansey E M. (eds) (2003) *Wellcome Witnesses to Twentieth Century Medicine*. Volume 16. London: The Wellcome Trust Centre for the History of Medicine at UCL, 94pp. ISBN 0 85484 088 5

Genetic testing
In: Christie D A, Tansey E M. (eds) (2003) *Wellcome Witnesses to Twentieth Century Medicine*. Volume 17. London: The Wellcome Trust Centre for the History of Medicine at UCL, 130pp. ISBN 0 85484 094 X

Foot and mouth disease: The 1967 outbreak and its aftermath
In: Reynolds L A, Tansey E M. (eds) (2003) *Wellcome Witnesses to Twentieth Century Medicine*. Volume 18. London: The Wellcome Trust Centre for the History of Medicine at UCL, 114pp. ISBN 0 85484 096 6

Environmental toxicology: The legacy of *Silent Spring*
In: Christie D A, Tansey E M. (eds) (2004) *Wellcome Witnesses to Twentieth Century Medicine*. Volume 19. London: The Wellcome Trust Centre for the History of Medicine at UCL, 132pp. ISBN 0 85484 091 5

Cystic fibrosis
In: Christie D A, Tansey E M. (eds) (2004) *Wellcome Witnesses to Twentieth Century Medicine*. Volume 20. London: The Wellcome Trust Centre for the History of Medicine at UCL, 120pp. ISBN 0 85484 086 9

Innovation in pain management
In: Reynolds L A, Tansey E M. (eds) (2004) *Wellcome Witnesses to Twentieth Century Medicine*. Volume 21. London: The Wellcome Trust Centre for the History of Medicine at UCL, 125pp. ISBN 0 85484 097 4

The Rhesus factor and disease prevention
In: Zallen D T, Christie D A, Tansey E M. (eds) (2004) *Wellcome Witnesses to Twentieth Century Medicine.* Volume 22. London: The Wellcome Trust Centre for the History of Medicine at UCL, 98pp. ISBN 0 85484 099 0

The recent history of platelets in thrombosis and other disorders
In: Reynolds L A, Tansey E M. (eds) (2005) *Wellcome Witnesses to Twentieth Century Medicine.* Volume 23. London: The Wellcome Trust Centre for the History of Medicine at UCL, 186pp. ISBN 0 85484 103 2

Short-course chemotherapy for tuberculosis
In: Christie D A, Tansey E M. (eds) (2005) *Wellcome Witnesses to Twentieth Century Medicine.* Volume 24. London: The Wellcome Trust Centre for the History of Medicine at UCL, 120pp. ISBN 0 85484 104 0

Prenatal corticosteroids for reducing morbidity and mortality after preterm birth
In: Reynolds L A, Tansey E M. (eds) (2005) *Wellcome Witnesses to Twentieth Century Medicine.* Volume 25. London: The Wellcome Trust Centre for the History of Medicine at UCL, 154pp. ISBN 0 85484 102 4

Public health in the 1980s and 1990s: Decline and rise?
In: Berridge V, Christie D A, Tansey E M. (eds) (2006) *Wellcome Witnesses to Twentieth Century Medicine.* Volume 26. London: The Wellcome Trust Centre for the History of Medicine at UCL, 101pp. ISBN 0 85484 106 7

Cholesterol, atherosclerosis and coronary disease in the UK, 1950–2000
In: Reynolds L A, Tansey E M. (eds) (2006) *Wellcome Witnesses to Twentieth Century Medicine.* Volume 27. London: The Wellcome Trust Centre for the History of Medicine at UCL, 164pp. ISBN 0 85484 107 5

Development of physics applied to medicine in the UK, 1945–90
In: Christie D A, Tansey E M. (eds) (2006) *Wellcome Witnesses to Twentieth Century Medicine.* Volume 28. The Wellcome Trust Centre for the History of Medicine at UCL, 141pp. ISBN 0 85484 108 3

Early development of total hip replacement
In: Reynolds L A, Tansey E M. (eds) (2007) *Wellcome Witnesses to Twentieth Century Medicine.* Volume 29. London: The Wellcome Trust Centre for the History of Medicine at UCL. This volume. ISBN 978 085484 111 0

The discovery, use and impact of platinum salts as chemotherapy agents for cancer
In: Christie D A, Tansey E M. (eds) (2007) *Wellcome Witnesses to Twentieth Century Medicine.* Volume 30. London: The Wellcome Trust Centre for the History of Medicine at UCL. In press. ISBN 978 085484 112 7

Hard copies of volumes 1–20 are now available for free, while stocks last. We would be happy to send complete sets to libraries in developing or restructuring countries. Available from Dr Carole Reeves at: *c.reeves@ucl.ac.uk*

All volumes are freely available online at www.ucl.ac.uk/histmed/ publications/wellcome-witnesses/index.html or by following the links to Publications/Wellcome Witnesses at www.ucl.ac.uk/histmed

A hard copy of volumes 21–29 can be ordered from www.amazon.co.uk; www.amazon.com; and all good booksellers for £6/$10 plus postage, using the ISBN.

Other publications

Technology transfer in Britain: The case of monoclonal antibodies
Tansey E M, Catterall P P. (1993) *Contemporary Record* 9: 409–44.

Monoclonal antibodies: A witness seminar on contemporary medical history
Tansey E M, Catterall P P. (1994) *Medical History* 38: 322–7.

Chronic pulmonary disease in South Wales coalmines: An eye-witness account of the MRC surveys (1937–42)
P D'Arcy Hart, edited and annotated by E M Tansey. (1998) *Social History of Medicine* 11: 459–68.

Ashes to Ashes – The history of smoking and health
Lock S P, Reynolds L A, Tansey E M. (eds) (1998) Amsterdam: Rodopi BV, 228pp. ISBN 90420 0396 0 (Hfl 125) (hardback). Reprinted 2003.

Witnessing medical history. An interview with Dr Rosemary Biggs
Professor Christine Lee and Dr Charles Rizza (interviewers). (1998)
Haemophilia **4**: 769–77.

**Witnessing the Witnesses: Pitfalls and potentials of the Witness Seminar
in twentieth century medicine**
By E M Tansey. In: Doel R, Soderqvist T. (eds) (2006) *Writing Recent
Science: The historiography of contemporary science, technology and medicine.*
London: Routledge, 260–78.

INTRODUCTION

This Witness Seminar adds an important oral history study to the many accounts of medical innovation that have appeared over the past 15 years.[2] This interest in innovations among historians, economists, sociologists and the general public can be explained by both the remarkable successes and the rising costs of medical technologies and drugs. Many recent studies have focused on the political, social and economic contexts as much as on the technologies themselves. In reconstructing these contexts, the recollections of the pioneers are invaluable (if not always indubitable). In this Witness Seminar some of the surviving actors involved in the early development of total hip replacement (THR) assembled to discuss their contributions and recollections. The resulting transcript provides an insight into the creation of a new medical technology in mid-twentieth-century Britain.

The THR operation has been seen as a landmark in twentieth-century surgery. Since the early 1960s it has played an important role in alleviating pain and restoring mobility to millions of people suffering from arthritic joints. Today about 35 000 hips are replaced in England and Wales each year by the NHS and many more operations are carried out in private hospitals.[3] THR has become one of the most commonly-performed elective surgical procedures worldwide. Its development was associated with innovation in materials, instruments, techniques and operative procedures, later adapted to treat other joints and applied across a range of surgical specialties. Hip replacement became a flagship operation and helped to raise the status of British orthopaedic surgery.[4]

The success of THR was not the result of one single breakthrough. Its origins lay in the interpositional- and hemi-arthroplasties developed between 1920 and 1950 in Europe and the US. The evolution of procedures for putting materials between the articulating surfaces or for replacing one side of the hip joint led

---

[2] See Pickstone (ed.) (1992); Löwy (ed.) (1993); Lawrence (ed.) (1994); Stanton (ed.) (2002); Webster (ed.) (2006); Timmermann and Anderson (eds) (2006).

[3] National Audit Office (2000).

[4] For a long-term analysis of what made orthopaedic surgery viable, from its foundation in the folk medicine traditions of bone setting in the eighteenth century to research-based practices and organized medical services in the twentieth century, see Pickstone (2006), 17–36.

to materials, designs and surgical techniques that proved crucial to its success.[5] However, THR was primarily a British innovation, one that started to take off in the late 1950s, under the NHS, but mainly in district general hospitals rather than in teaching hospitals. It was created in hospital units at Norwich, Wrightington (near Wigan), Stanmore, Redhill and later Exeter.[6]

The story begins with the pioneering operations of Philip Wiles at the Middlesex Hospital in the late 1930s;[7] it continues through the later work of his registrar G Kenneth McKee at the Norfolk and Norwich Hospital, and includes the programmes at the other centres, led by John Charnley (Wrightington), John Scales and 'Ginger' Wilson (Stanmore), Peter Ring (Redhill) and Robin Ling and Clive Lee (Exeter).

The aim of the Witness Seminar was to reveal some of the personal stories and relationships behind the published accounts. Though many of the early innovators are no longer with us, their tales live on through the reminiscences of their trainees and some of the nurses, surgeons, engineers and manufacturers who were involved with the original centres and with later developments, who spoke at this meeting. The transcript shows early THR as classic British postwar science, characterized by improvisation, ingenuity, long hours and low budgets. But by the 1970s THRs were taken up across the Western world, and by the 1990s the British companies had become attractive acquisitions for healthcare corporations. The global market is now dominated by a handful of multinational

---

[5] In the US, for instance, Dr Marius Smith-Petersen experimented with a number of materials in the 1930s (including glass and Pyrex) for his interpositional cup arthroplasty until he had some success with Vitallium® (a chrome–cobalt alloy) [see Figure 12 and Appendix 3]. This alloy was used by Drs Fred Thompson and Austin Moore for their hemi-arthroplasties to replace the head of the femur in the early 1950s. These prostheses had an advantage over earlier hemi-arthroplasties, fixed with plates and screws on the outside of the femur, because their stems, which went down the medullary canal, were more stable. They were also much more reliable than the acrylic polyethylene hemi-arthroplasty developed by the Judet brothers in France in the late 1940s, which only had a small stem. See note 96 and Appendix 3, pages 101–06.

[6] For detailed histories of THR and its precursors from the point of view of the development of materials, see: Parsons (1972); and Walker (1977): 253–75. For a chronological history based around solutions, see Scales (1966–7). For a more recent historical overview, see Klenerman (2002): 13–23.

[7] Thermistokles Glück (1853–1942) replaced a number of tuberculosis-damaged joints with ivory prostheses, which were fixed with a bone glue composed of colophony or rosin, pumice powder, and plaster of Paris in the 1880s. These may have included an ivory total hip replacement, but his work was discredited when he was forced to retract his results after an argument with Professor Ernst von Bergman (1836–1907), his boss and head of the Berlin surgical clinic. See Glück (1891). See also www.totaljoints.info/Prehistory_GluckPean.htm (visited 2 November 2006).

companies, mostly based in the US, some of which are associated with the pharmaceutical giants.

The early development of THR was a 'cottage industry', in which surgeon–inventors with a knowledge of engineering principles worked with craft-based technicians, university departments and small surgical instrument manufacturers. For instance, in the late 1950s John Charnley employed the technician Harry Craven to work from the workshop at Charnley's home, making Teflon® acetabular cups and finishing forged stainless steel femoral prostheses on a lathe. These would be sterilized in formaldehyde overnight ready for operating the next day.[8] Charnley had liaised with the Engineering Department at UMIST over materials for the prosthesis and with the Victoria University of Manchester Dental School over the pink, acrylic dental cement that he used to fix his prostheses in place (see pages 13 and 22). He worked with the Leeds-based surgical instrument company Chas F Thackray to forge his femoral prosthesis and by 1963 they were mass-producing his prosthesis at their factory.[9] Throughout the 1960s Charnley also worked with another local company to develop a clean air operating theatre environment to reduce post-operative infections, which were ruining nearly 10 per cent of his hip replacement operations. This Bolton-based company, Howorth Air Conditioning, had been developing clean air environments for cotton mills and breweries since the late nineteenth century and adapted their technologies to Charnley's needs.[10]

This use of local companies and expertise was a feature of all of the five early THR centres.[11] But each leading surgeon used the particular surgical approach he had learned for earlier hip operations, including tumours, fractured necks of femur etc. [see Figure 24]. Their choice of materials also varied considerably (stainless steel, cobalt–chrome alloy, Teflon®, and high-density polyethylene), as did the prosthesis design (femoral head size and neck, stem and cup geometry)

---

[8] For an account of Charnley's research including the early setup for manufacturing prostheses by hand, see Waugh (1990): 116–17. See also note 7, page 7.

[9] For the Thackray company's relationship with Charnley, see Wainwright (1997): 73–105, especially Chapters 9 and 10.

[10] See Howorth (2002); and Whyte (2001): 9–20, especially Chapter 2.

[11] It is interesting to note their ingenuity in adapting materials and existing technologies from the aircraft, dental prosthetic and surgical-instrument industries to their purposes. For example, many of the early biomechanical engineers came from the aircraft industry, which was a rich source of research on corrosion-resistant materials, and the use of chrome–cobalt alloys and acrylic cement was well established in dental prosthetics. See Professors Swanson on pages 26–28 and Dowson on pages 28–30.

and the methods of fixation (screws or nails, acrylic cement and bone in-growth). These local variations led to a plethora of debates about the best mode of THR; the arguments continued at formal meetings and in more informal settings like the annual orthopaedic skiing trip to the Alps.[12]

This transcript is also a testament to why these debates continue to the present day, and to the shifting concerns about the body's reactions to materials and cement, which made certain combinations of materials and fixation methods more attractive at particular stages in the development of THR. For instance, concerns about the effect of the debris produced by metal-on-metal articulations promoted a general shift in the early 1970s to cemented metal-on-plastic hips, especially after the very good early results with the Charnley prosthesis. But towards the end of that decade, new worries about the biocompatibility of the cement and the effect of polyethylene wear particles led to a resurgence of metal-on-metal combinations. Later problems with the fixation of metal-on-metal components, especially those using new bioactive coating methods (like hydroxyapatite), made metal-on-plastic attractive again, and in the 1990s more accurate machining techniques created the possibility of obtaining good results from metal-on-metal hip resurfacing.[13] For over 50 years now, the debates have continued, partly because of continual novelties, but also because the results are hard to predict and can only be judged over 10–20 years. Short-term studies can only pick up serious failures, and records of long-term performance are less complete than they might have been. The transcript shows how proposals to create a British register of hip implants in the 1980s came to little.[14]

The seminar participants also considered the attempts to impose standards on the design and manufacture of hip prostheses. The 1970s and 1980s saw little consensus in the committees set up in Britain and Europe. Standardization and regulation in Britain came much later than in the US: the Medical Devices

---

[12] For a description of the British Orthopaedic Ski Group, see Waugh (1990): 93; 130–1. Its name was later changed to Study Group (BSOG) and is used throughout the transcript.

[13] Hip resurfacing was attempted by Charnley in the late 1950s with a PTFE double cup (see Figure 4) and Freeman in the early 1970s with a metal-on-polyethylene combination (see Figure 18). There were early failures, but the Birmingham metal-on-metal hip resurfacing, developed in the 1990s (see Appendix 3, page 106) was widely copied and resurfacing is now a common operation for younger patients, see page 32.

[14] For instance, the recommendations of the DoH Implant Advisory Group [see pages 39–41 and Sweetnam (1981)]. Although hip registers were set up in Scandinavia in the period, the Swedish National Hip Arthroplasty Register had begun collecting and analysing data about all primary total hip replacements and re-operations and revisions of hip implants in 1979, while the Norwegian Arthroplasty Register was started in 1987.

Agency (MDA) was not formed until the 1990s and it was then merged with the Medicines Control Agency (MCA) in 2003 to form the Medicines and Healthcare products Regulatory Agency (MHRA).[15] In the early period of THR in the UK, as covered by this seminar, single-centre follow-up studies were the best data available. Regional registers began to appear in Britain in the 1990s and in April 2003 the National Joint Registry for England and Wales (NJR) was set up.[16] Recently, as in some other countries, the National Institute for Clinical Excellence (NICE) has produced studies of the cost effectiveness of prostheses based on long-term follow-up studies.[17] These studies clearly show that the most common and most reliable of the models used in Britain are closely related to the Charnley designs of the 1960s.

THR materials and techniques came to be adapted for a greater range of types of patient and for the replacement of other joints; they proved to be the basis of a huge global industry that now has many of the characteristics of the pharmaceutical business, including 'me too' models and huge amounts of money spent to secure 'surgeon loyalty'. It is a far cry from the British pioneers of the 1950s and 1960s who worked in the NHS, led the collaborations with engineers and companies, and achieved long-lasting results with remarkable economy. To them, millions of older (and some younger) people now owe substantial enhancements in their quality of life. This transcript will serve as a permanent record of the early developments and we are most grateful to all who took part.

Francis Neary and John Pickstone,
Centre for the History of Science, Technology and Medicine,
University of Manchester

---

[15] See their website at www.mhra.gov.uk (visited 2 November 2006).

[16] The latest NJR report for 2005/06 records 82 per cent of the hip and knee operations performed in England and Wales and can be viewed at www.njrcentre.org.uk/Public/PPEhomepage.htm (visited 12 December 2006).

[17] For instance, NICE (2000): 1–9. See www.nice.org.uk/page.aspx?o=510 for later guidelines to the NHS and for patients, freely available (visited 2 November 2006).

EARLY DEVELOPMENT OF
TOTAL HIP REPLACEMENT

The transcript of a Witness Seminar held by the Wellcome Trust Centre for the History of Medicine at UCL, London, on 14 March 2006

Edited by L A Reynolds and E M Tansey

EARLY DEVELOPMENT OF TOTAL HIP REPLACEMENT

Participants

Professor Sir Christopher Booth
Lady Charnley
Mr Tristram Charnley
Mr Harry Craven[†]
Ms Clare Darrah
Mr Graham Deane
Professor Duncan Dowson
Mrs Sheila Edwards
Mr Reg Elson
Dr Alex Faulkner
Professor Michael Freeman
Mrs Phyllis Hampson
Mr Kevin Hardinge
Mr Mike Heywood-Waddington
Mr Geoff King
Mr John Kirkup

Mr Krishna (Ravi) Kunzru
Miss Betty Lee
Mr Alan Lettin (Chair)
Dr Francis Neary
Mr John Older
Professor John Pickstone
Mr John Read
Mr Peter Ring
Mr Ian Stephen
Mr Malcolm Swann
Professor Alan Swanson
Sir Rodney Sweetnam
Mr Keith Tucker
Mr Victor Wheble
Mr Michael Wilson
Professor B Michael Wroblewski

Among those attending the meeting: Mrs Jan Sherwood, Professor John Walker-Smith, Mr Nigel Wheble

Apologies include: Mr Ron Ansell, Mr Frank Brown, Mr John Challis, Mr Simon Chaplin, Mr Chris Faux, Professor John Fisher, Mr Graham Gie, Mr Barry Hinves, Mr Frank Horan, Dr M F Leclerc, Dr Clive Lee, Mr Ian Leslie, Professor Robin Ling, Professor Archie Malcolm, Mr Derek McMinn, Professor Colin Normand, Professor John Paul, Mr James Scott, Dr Jean Smellie, Mr Richard Todd, Mr Roger Vickers, Mr J N (Ginger) Wilson[‡]

[†]Died 16 February 2007

[‡]Died 2 March 2006

Dr Daphne Christie: We are very grateful to our advisers, Ravi Kunzru and Francis Neary, for their help with the organization of the meeting and I am particularly grateful to Alan Lettin, who has kindly agreed to chair the meeting this afternoon. So, without further ado, I will pass you over to the Chairman.

Mr Alan Lettin:[1] Thank you very much. These Witness Seminars have been going since 1993.[2] It strikes me that perhaps it is about 20 years too late for one on total hip replacement [THR, also known as total hip arthroplasty, THA, see Figure 1], because if one had been held 20 years ago, the modern innovators would have been here in person. In fact, one or two are here, I am looking straight at Peter Ring. I think the concept of this meeting started with Ravi Kunzru, who has become very interested in medical history since retiring as a Consultant Orthopaedic Surgeon, and Francis Neary and his boss, John Pickstone, who is a professor of medical history at the University of Manchester.

I think most people would know that the idea of replacing diseased and damaged joints by artificial implants was not new in the 1950s when John Charnley and Ken McKee and others really put joint replacement on the map. People tried in the nineteenth century, in the great explosion of surgical knowledge and effort at the end of that century, but for all intents and purposes, we will be talking about the second half of the twentieth century, a period which began with John Charnley and Ken McKee and perhaps ended 20 years later with Michael Freeman and the double cup.[3] Everything since then has been a variation on a theme and what we really want, in the absence of those early innovators, is for the people here, who have been asked to come because they worked with or for those pioneers, to reminisce and to tell us what happened.

Although I said that it really started with McKee and Charnley, I think perhaps we should pay some tribute to Philip Wiles [Figure 2], who, as I understand it, did the first total hip replacement in 1938 [see Appendix 3, page 101].

Sir Rodney Sweetnam was Philip Wiles' houseman, registrar, and succeeded him at the Middlesex Hospital, London. I thought it would be appropriate if Sir Rodney started the ball rolling. If everybody in this room speaks, they are

---

[1] Biographical notes appear on pages 133–45.

[2] For the background to the Witness Seminar as an historical tool, see pages xi–xxiii.

[3] The Imperial College London Hospital (ICLH) hip replacement, see Figure 18. See also Brigitte and Earl (2006); Padgett *et al.* (2006); Parker and Gurusamy (2006).

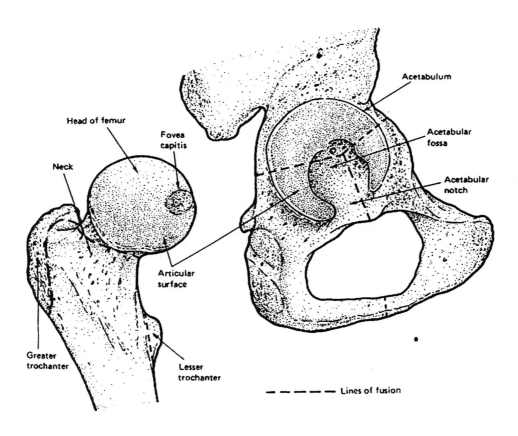

Figure 1: The disarticulated hip joint, the site of a total hip replacement.
L: the head of the femur; R: the acetabulum, part of the pelvis.

only going to be able to do so for four minutes each, so we don't really want anyone speaking for longer than four minutes at a time anyway. Of course, there shouldn't be any undue constraints, but I do beg you not to take the floor for too long. Rodney, I am sure you will set a tremendous example to everyone by telling us about Philip Wiles' contribution.

Sir Rodney Sweetnam: Yes, and I will do it in three and half minutes. Thank you very much and thank you for asking me. You made it sound as though there was a degree of nepotism, Chairman. Yes, I was Philip Wiles' houseman, and I did indeed succeed him, although I wasn't his registrar.

I want to draw everybody's attention to the pioneer work that my ex-chief and predecessor [see Figure 2] did, and, to that end, on your chairs, is a copy of a paper in the *British Journal of Surgery* that he wrote in 1958, describing his first attempt at a total hip replacement arthroplasty. You will see that in the right-hand column on the first page, he describes what I believe to be the first total hip replacement [in the UK] in 1938, at the Middlesex Hospital, replacing the socket and the femoral component.[4]

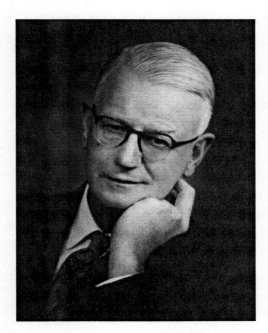

Figure 2: Mr Philip Wiles FRCS, *c.* 1950.

---

[4] Wiles (1958). See Appendix 3, page 101.

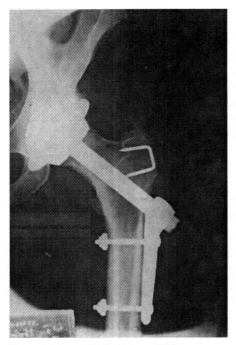

Figure 3: X-ray of Wiles' hip, c. 1950s.

He describes animal experimentation, and later the insertion of six of these prostheses into patients. He also goes on to say that he had no adequate follow-up, as the war intervened and, of the six patients, he only knew of one later. That one patient became my patient when I succeeded him in 1960. That patient had a painful, stiff, but slightly mobile hip, which was the site of one of Wiles' six total joint replacements. I removed the artificial joint and, if I remember correctly, arthrodesed the hip – I may have done a Girdlestone, I can't remember.[5] But the prosthesis is now in the archives of the British Orthopaedic Association (BOA), on loan to the Hunterian Museum at the Royal College of Surgeons. This first attempt at total hip replacement had some similarity to the present-day, so-called 'surface' replacement [see Appendix 3, page 106].

In my time Philip Wiles was a modest man, you'll see that in his paper he makes relatively short reference to this major contribution in hip surgery worldwide – six cases, he dismisses it, goes on to describe all the other operations.

---

[5] A Girdlestone operation is a resection arthroplasty of the hip, removing the head and neck of the femur, which usually leaves the patient with a pain-free hip. The femur is left loose allowing some movement between it and the acetabulum (pelvis) – a 'pseudoarthrosis' or false joint. See the Glossary, page 148.

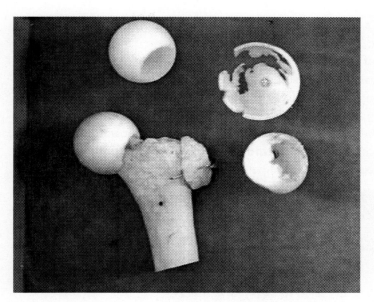

Figure 4: Charnley PTFE double cup implant, c. 1960.

Lettin: I suppose, having said that very few of the originators are left, Peter Ring is here. Peter, I don't know whether you could perhaps tell us the sequence of events? Was it McKee who produced the first total hip replacement, or was it John Charnley, or was it even you? I know it wasn't the Stanmore.[6]

Mr Peter Ring: No, it certainly wasn't me. I was a registrar at the time when John Charnley was working with PTFE [polytetrafluoroethylene (Teflon®, Fluon®)],[7] and later I became a consultant at Redhill and went to a meeting two or three years later, at which both McKee and Charnley were present, one demonstrating the metal-on-plastic hip and the other the metal-on-metal.[8]

---

[6] McKee produced an all-metal prototype replacement joint in 1940, although his results were not published until 1951 [McKee (1951)], the Judet brothers inserted a perspex femoral head in 1946 [Judet and Judet (1950)], and the Charnley hip was the first total hip replacement system to be adopted worldwide. Foreman-Peck (1995): 109. See Appendix 3, pages 101–06, for illustrations of the cups and stems mentioned in this transcript and the materials used.

[7] Teflon® is the trade name for a family of PTFE resins produced by DuPont, Wilmington, Delaware, USA. Charnley's acetabular and femoral components were made from Fluon® resin produced by Imperial Chemical Industries (ICI) in the UK. Charnley (1974) describes the material illustrated in Figure 4 as polytef. Many participants called this Teflon® during the meeting, which has been replaced in the text with the more accurate term PTFE. See Li and Burstein (1994).

[8] See note 42.

It occurred to me that they were both making a rather simple job difficult by using bone cement,[9] which was a relatively untried material at that time. And since we had a prosthesis at that time, Moore's,[10] which gave a reasonable result, certainly in the treatment of fractures of the hip joint, if one could match that to some sort of cup that was fixed firmly, you might avoid the use of bone cement [see Figure 5]. I had spent two or three years demonstrating anatomy before that, and one of the areas that was quite obvious to an anatomist was the ileopubic bar of bone. And as an orthopaedic surgeon, I became familiar with this in doing arthrodesis, because one attempted to get the trifin nail up the

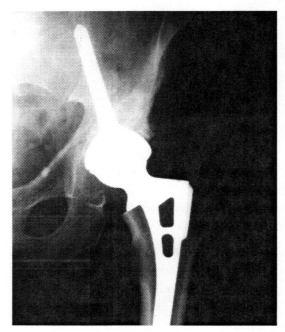

Figure 5: The Ring total hip replacement: X-ray of THR in position, 1970.

[9] Charnley describes the properties of polymethylmethacrylate (PMMA), the self-curing bone cement: 'PMMA for orthopaedic usage (for example, CMW [see Appendix 2]) is packaged as two components: 20ml of liquid and 40g of powder. The liquid contains the PMMA monomer, stabilizer and activator. The powder contains the polymer, a radio-opaque substance and polymerization initiators. When added together and mixed, polymerization occurs. At first the cement is a relatively low viscosity glistening paste. The viscosity of the preparation steadily increases and the surface becomes dull. The rapid final phase of polymerization is associated with an exothermic reaction. The material then becomes a solid resin. When used in large volumes, a bulk state, PMMA behaves in a different way from the thin mantle seen in prosthetic fixation.' McCaskie *et al.* (1998): 37. See also Charnley (1970) and note 37.

[10] See Appendix 3, page 102.

ileopubic bar of bone for secure fixation. It seemed, therefore, that if you could locate a cup with a long screw thread up the ileopubic bar of the bone, you could hope for a reasonably sound method of fixation. If you also got a cup that was orientated more or less directly, and certainly uniformly, and matched that to a femoral component and you had a total hip replacement [see Figure 5]. For the development of that, I am very indebted to Maurice Down,[11] who put the resources of his firm at my disposal and helped me in its development, as he did for a number of orthopaedic surgeons.

Lettin: Essentially, what you were developing was an uncemented implant, because you didn't feel that cement was the way forward; was that the essence of your contribution? Now, obviously, we have asked one or two people along who were associated with the early development, including John Kirkup, who worked as a junior with McKee [Figure 6]. Perhaps you could tell us, John, what went on way back in the early days?

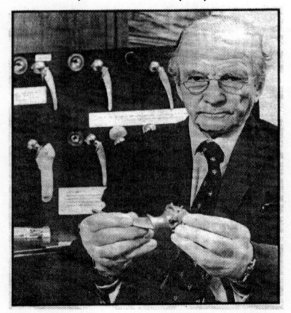

Figure 6: Ken McKee with his total hip replacement system. Reproduced by permission of the ©Eastern Evening News.

---

[11] Mr Maurice Down OBE was Chairman and Managing Director of the small medical equipment firm, Downs Surgical Ltd, Mitcham, Surrey, that manufactured and marketed the Ring THR from 1964. Mr Peter Ring wrote: 'Maurice Down remained until the firm was eventually taken over by Smith's Industries in the mid-1980s, although it continued to manufacture my implants and continued the trading name of Downs for many years after that'. Letter to Mrs Lois Reynolds, 17 October 2006.

Mr John Kirkup: I had the privilege of being there with Ken McKee from 1956 to 1958, six months as a senior house officer (SHO) and 18 months as a registrar, and the thing that struck me was that he was not just an orthopaedic surgeon of mechanical bent, but he was a general orthopaedist, with his clinics full of interesting material, a fact that converted me to orthopaedic surgery. But there was no doubt that he was interested in hips, perhaps because his clinics were full of farmers and farm workers, who were otherwise very fit, except for an arthritic hip, or an arthritic knee, or both. And this was one of the things that motivated him towards that particular field of surgery, which he started in 1951, you may remember. The first hip in stainless steel was unsatisfactory, as was the second; the third, in the alloy of chrome and cobalt, lasted some three years.[12] When I arrived in 1956, he was starting what he called Mark 3 hips, comprising metal-to-metal chrome–cobalt, with a flanged acetabulum, in the centre of which were three holes with three screws. I thought this was rather unsatisfactory, but anyway, the operation worked [for an X-ray of a later version, see Figure 7].

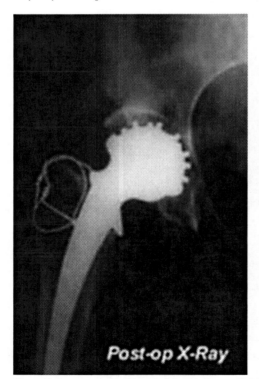

Figure 7: Post-operative X-ray of the McKee artificial joint, 1963.

---

[12] McKee (1953).

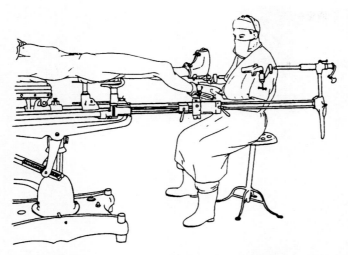

Figure 8: Hawley orthopaedic table showing a non-sterile assistant controlling the leg.

It was interesting. One day he said, 'We are replacing a hip tomorrow', and as I was a bit late getting to the theatre that morning, I saw him going up the steps rubbing something on the back of his right buttock, and then saw this was a prosthesis. He said, 'Yes, we must ensure that we have complete slipperiness, it's very important that we reduce the friction'. It was the hip ball he had polished in his workshop the night before. Anyway, the fact is that this somewhat odd operation appeared to work. You had to have the patient on a Hawley table [Figure 8] and Frank, the orthopaedic technician, was called upon to move the leg as necessary at the relevant moment.[13] The patient remained in bed for ten or 12 days, until the wound was healed, and stayed in hospital for maybe three or four weeks.

For many patients this surgery succeeded; I saw them at follow-up and most were very pleased. However, McKee was only doing something like ten a year. And then in 1960, of course, he was converted to the use of cement.[14]

Lettin: That leads us on very nicely, I suppose, to John Read. There are several people here, not least Lady Charnley, who were associated with Sir John [Charnley]. Of course, John, you were working for him fairly early on. What are your recollections? I think it's quite clear that Sir John introduced cement into the operation.

---

[13] See Figure 8 for an example of a Hawley table.

[14] McKee and Watson-Farrar (1966).

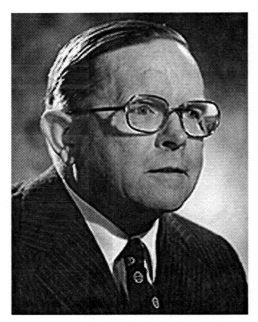

Figure 9: Professor Sir John Charnley FRCS FRS[15]

Mr John Read: I arrived at Wrightington[16] in 1961, having previously done three years as a registrar at Sunderland Orthopaedic and Accident Hospital. Before my arrival, John Charnley [Figure 9] had been working on his artificial hip using a PTFE socket and a stainless steel femoral head. Actually, the first one he produced was a double PTFE cup [see Figure 4], which was a failure, and after that he moved on to using a metal femoral head. And the initial results of that had been quite good, but there were several problems. One was that, within a year, PTFE was beginning to show signs of wear, and the other was that he had a high infection rate,[17] because at his unit at Wrightington, he'd been allocated, I think, ten theatre hours altogether, but the theatre was very basic – it didn't have a recognizable ventilating system, was used by all sorts of people, at all sorts of times, and it had a high infection rate, which I think was about 7 per cent.[18]

---

[15] Professor Mike Wroblewski wrote: 'Charnley gave this photo, autographed, to his past Residents.' Note on draft transcript, 24 October 2006.

[16] The Centre for Hip Surgery at Wrightington Hospital, near Manchester.

[17] Charnley and Eftekhar (1969); Charnley (1972).

[18] Professor Mike Wroblewski wrote: 'The infection rate before clean air enclosure was 8.9 per cent'. Note on draft transcript, 20 June 2006. See Charnley and Eftekhar (1969): 645; also Figures 12, 13 and 24.

Before I arrived he started designing his greenhouse, to produce his own fresh air inflow from outside, and Harry Craven [Figure 10], who is here today, built the enclosure in his workshop.[19] My first theatre list was with this greenhouse being used for the first time, which was quite something. I am sure you have all seen pictures of it from time to time [Figures 12 and 13]. It only took the patient's body. The anaesthetist was kept outside, because he was dirty anyway, but we had windows at the side so that other people could look in and see what was going on.

Lettin: One of the topics that we want to get to is infection and the question of the greenhouse might be better discussed then. Was that your main recollection? What about the cement? Was that introduced in your time, or before?

Read: A little before, I think, and the cement that we used initially still had the pink dental dye in it, which was quite useful actually because you could see where it was going quite well.[20]

Lettin: Mr Craven, would you like to comment on those early times?

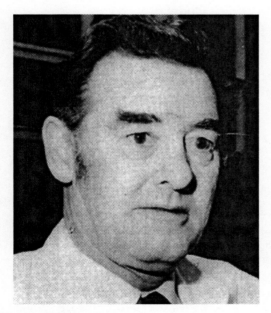

Figure 10: Harry Craven, 1981.

---

[19] Anonymous (1960); Lowbury and Lidwell (1978); Johnston (1981); Bintcliffe (1983).

[20] Mr John Read wrote: 'Dental acrylic with a pink dye to match the gums'. Note on draft transcript, 4 July 2006.

Mr Harry Craven: Speaking of the cement, I think we started using it about 1960. This was when we were still on with the PTFE and then we went on to other stuff called Fluorosint®[21] – funny name, and funny mixture – and we didn't do very many with that. But I designed another hip, which I thought was a three-dimensional hip, where you had a Smith-Petersen cup [Figure 11][22] and a plastic socket put inside it, cemented in with the acrylic cement, and then you got the main head of the prosthesis going into the main HDP socket. I thought if there's any movement, you'd get three movements, which could help the life of the hip socket.

Apparently this wasn't so, although some of the chaps at Wrightington – Kirk Houston was one – loved doing these, after we had gone on to the high-density polyethylene (HDP). John Charnley said to him: 'I don't want you to do those, I want you to do research on them'. But Kirk Houston still insisted on doing them.

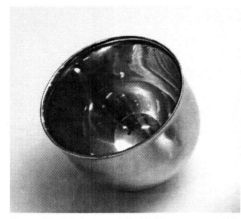

Figure 11: Stainless steel Smith-Petersen cup (4.5cm diameter x 4cm), c. 1938.

---

[21] Charnley used Fluorosint®, a mica-reinforced Teflon®, for the cups. The replacement UHMWPE [Hoechst, Oberhausen, Germany] had been used in the European textile industry in the 1950s for impact bearings of mechanical looms. Charnley's first UHMWPE socket, labelled RCH 1000, was implanted in November 1962. [Gomez and Morcuende (2005b): 33; Charnley (1979): 87–9, Figure 6.29.] Professor Mike Wroblewski wrote: 'The Press-Fit cup was used from 1962/3 to 1965; 336 were implanted. It was not used after 1965. The longest surviving, well-functioning press-fit is in a patient aged 44 at the time of surgery. He has now completed 42 years of clinical success. This is the longest surviving, well-functioning THA.' Note on draft transcript, 24 October 2006. Freeman *et al.* (1985); Swanson and Evarts (1984). See also Semlitsch and Willert (1997): 73.

[22] Smith-Petersen (1939); Berntsen and Bertelsen (1952).

With regard to the greenhouse [see Figure 12], it was built in 1960, and this was done, as John [Read] said, because things weren't sterile. I managed to get a little ventilation unit, which was put outside the enclosure and we had the greenhouse [see also Figure 13]. John Charnley used to come for me on a Sunday, and say: 'Can you come down for half an hour?', and it would last all day. We would do smoke tests in the theatre, all kinds of tests, to see where the air was going. And we ended up with two bags inside it, which were filters, but the unit I got had six filters inside it with two micron filters [see Figure 14] and, from then on, the infection rate seemed to drop.[23] The people who had lent me the sterile unit, which was outside the ventilation plant, was the firm of Howorths.[24] It was a friend of John Charnley who put me on to them. The chief engineer, a Mr Poulton, came out and I showed him what I wanted, and he lent me this ventilation plant, and then he phoned me and asked for Mr Howorth to come. And it was a bit of a laugh really. He came in an E-type Jag – you needed

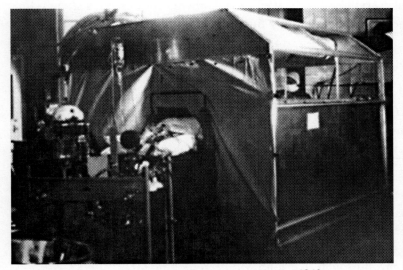

Figure 12: Charnley's original greenhouse clean air enclosure, 1960.

---

[23] Charnley's greenhouse succeeded in reducing the sepsis rate in THR operations from 8.9 per cent in 1960 to 0.9 per cent in 1968. Lowbury and Lidwell (1978): 800. See also Anonymous (1976); Howorth (1985); Berg *et al.* (1991).

[24] Mr F N Howorth represented his air filtration firm, Howorth Surgicair, from Bolton, Lancashire [established in 1854, known as Howorth Airtech Ltd in 1996] that had originally designed filters for brewers and pharmaceutical manufacturers to remove particles, or bacteria, from the air. See Scottish Society for Contamination Control (S2C2) (2004a and b), in particular (2004a): 4–5 for photographs of the 1962 greenhouse and a later undated commercially-available model [s2c2@mech.gla.ac.uk]. See also page 80.

a shoe horn to get in – and he introduced himself to me, and I took him in theatre, got him gowned up, and said, 'You can watch the operations through the windows'. He looked through the windows and collapsed on the floor: it took three of us to drag him out.

And then the hip success rate improved and we, or rather I, got the HDP from West Germany through a sales technician who came. I asked if he could give me a piece – he was trying to sell things – as I wanted to put it under test. I had built a test rig for testing all the materials we could get on a flat surface, and he sent me a piece. I got all the information on it as well from West Germany, and I tested it. John [Charnley] was going away to Zurich, I think it was, for about three weeks, and he came in and said, 'What are you testing?' I replied, 'Polyethylene'. 'Throw the bloody stuff away,' he said, 'it's no good'. Anyway, I carried on testing it, and when he came back he asked what I was testing and I said, 'The stuff you told me to throw away'. He asked for my graph, because I did a graph of everything I did. 'Well', I said, 'there's your graph, a straight line all around the room and, from my figures, I have calculated that it would last 70 years'.[25]

I don't know what the record is at the moment with regard to hip joints, but on a flat surface, I got 70 years work out of it.[26]

Lettin: Lady Charnley, do you have any recollections, I am sure you have lots of recollections.

Lady Charnley: I certainly don't want to hold the floor for any length of time, partly because I am having great difficulty in speaking today with a peculiar throat. But yes, of course, I have very many marvellous memories, and I must say that it was Harry Craven's persistence in doing what he shouldn't have done, to put this piece of high-density polyethylene on the wear-testing machine that he had made at the hospital, against John's wishes, which of course eventually was the great breakthrough that John had been looking for.[27]

---

[25] Charnley (1974): 1028.

[26] See, for example, Wroblewski (1997). Professor Mike Wroblewski wrote: 'I have an original specimen from 1962.' Note on draft transcript, 20 June 2006.

[27] For a remark on Mr Harry Craven's testing of the HDP samples and a full discussion of the progression from a large-diameter 41mm Thompson or Austin Moore prosthesis to the Charnley low-friction arthroplasty using the 22.225mm head, see Charnley (1974):1027–8. Early prostheses were tested on hand-made wear-test machines. Modern testing equipment can be seen at www.dur.ac.uk/cbme/facilities/ (visited 21 September 2006).

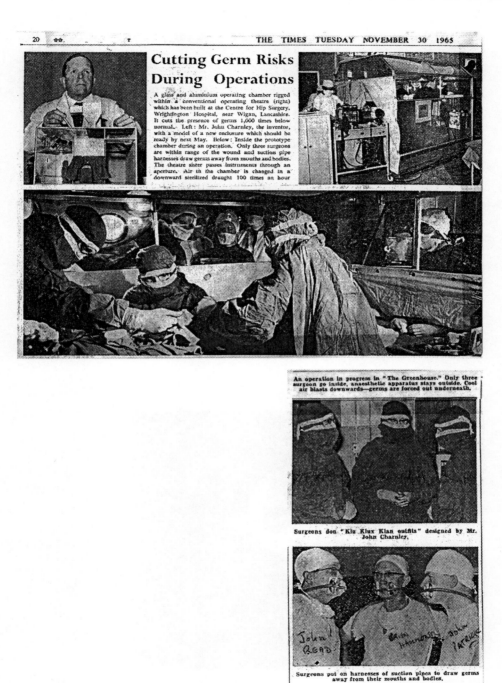

Figure 13: Filters and masks: cutting infection rates. From *The Times* (30 November 1965): 20.
Provided and annotated by Mr John Read.

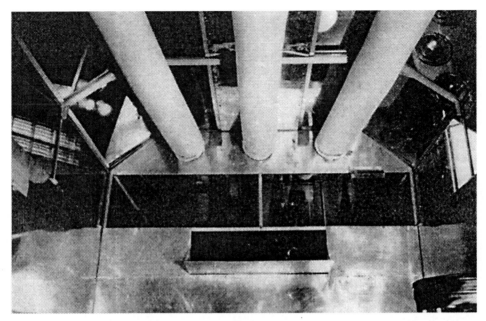

Figure 14: Looking down on to the greenhouse roof showing three cloth infuser bags inflated with clean air.

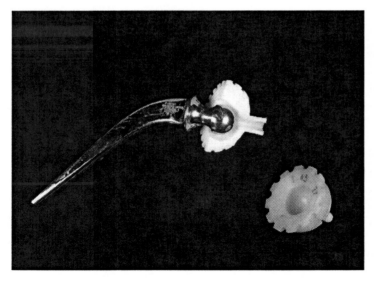

Figure 15: The Charnley low-friction arthroplasty in use from November 1962, having a thick socket of UHMWPE with deep external serrations and a small femoral-head on the flat-back prosthesis.

At that time, John was extremely despondent. He had a great many patients who initially had done incredibly well with the PTFE, and when the PTFE cups began to wear he had nightmares. In fact, I know it is well documented that he used to wake up at about 3 o'clock in the morning and I would see him with his head in his hands, saying, 'I don't know what I am going to do with all the patients that are going wrong'. But, of course, when HDP came and was proved to be a very hard-wearing material, he was able to operate on all the patients who had had PTFE and, of course, that was the start of the great breakthrough in hip replacement [Figure 15]. I could go on all afternoon, but I shall happily hand over to somebody else.

Lettin: Thank you very much for those recollections. Now I know that the Stanmore total hip replacement came a bit after the McKee and the Charnley. We haven't really decided which came first, but we've decided that Wiles really has precedence in the introduction of total hip replacement. I do know that Stanmore came a bit later.[28] Unfortunately, 'Ginger' Wilson [Figure 16], who was due to talk about the early Stanmore experience, passed away a couple of weeks ago, but his daughter and son are both here. I don't know if they would like to say anything.[29]

Mrs Sheila Edwards: We can only tell you silly stories, having lived with the Stanmore through our formative years. I know nothing really practical about it, I think Phyllis [Hampson] will be able to tell you much more about it than I can.

We do have recollections of mother's tablespoons going missing from the kitchen drawer, to be used as some sort of reamer, or battered into some shape he needed. There was another ghastly story about something exploding in theatre and leaving ball bearings all over the theatre floor.[30] We are not quite sure what that was. We are grateful that you have invited us here today to stand up for him.

---

[28] Duff-Barclay *et al.* (1966); Scales and Wilson (1969); Wilson and Scales (1973).

[29] See Owen (2006). Mr Michael Wilson wrote: 'He inserted the first Stanmore total hip on 25 April 1963 with John Scales, and afterwards initiated the Bone Tumour Registry. He described Wilson's operation for hallux valgus, but gained media attention from his descriptions of "Winkle-Picker's Disease" and "The Battered Buttock". I've just checked my Father's diary for 25 April 1963. He wrote: "Did our first Scales–Wilson prosthesis. It went very well – took about three hours, but this was mainly because we went very slowly and took lots of photos. I can hardly believe it was so easy. Now it depends upon healing and rehab".' E-mail to Mrs Lois Reynolds, 17 October 2006.

[30] See note 86. See also an example of a reamer in Figure 22, page 39.

Lettin: I think we are probably coming to the end of this initial topic and, as I believe I said, we thought that perhaps the final innovation, if you like, was the double cup. Everything since then has been a variation on a theme.

The conventional total joint replacement has had, for example, hydroxyapatite surfaces and various other modifications, but essentially the basic design remains the same. But the double cup, I think, is obviously something quite different. Michael [Freeman], would you like to say why and how you came to do it, and why Derek McMinn's resurfacing arthroplasty seemed to work and yours didn't.[31]

Professor Michael Freeman: The concept of a two-part resurfacing arthroplasty, I dare say, came from a number of people, but the reason it came to me was made up of two things: one was that the early results of conventional THR, I won't go into details, were not absolutely wonderful technically, and there were some particularly dramatic failures on the femoral side in the hands of both my colleagues and myself. It seemed a pity to treat a disease that was only a few millimetres thick on the femoral side, with an operation that ended with approximately one-third of the femur being severely damaged. That was one factor. The other was that one of my senior colleagues, Scottie Law, had a very large experience of single cup arthroplasty, having been in the US, in

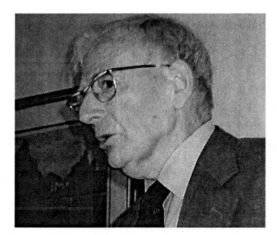

Figure 16: Mr 'Ginger' Wilson, *c.* 2000.

---

[31] Derek McMinn reintroduced the double cup or 'resurfacing arthroplasty' with his own design at the Royal Orthopaedic Hospital, Birmingham, in 1991. McMinn *et al.* (1996). See also note 118 and Appendix 3, page 106.

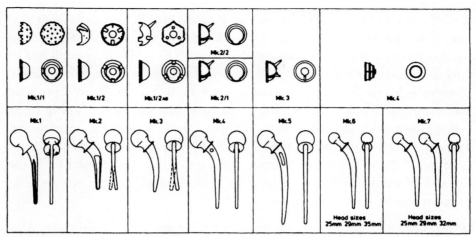

Figure 17: Principal stages in the design and development of the Stanmore prosthesis, 1960–85. Note that the first four models were double, with the base secured to the acetabulum and the inner cup rotating inside.

Boston, after the war, and it was a very small step to think that you could cement the metal component to the femur and a polyethylene socket to the acetabulum. The man who actually designed the [ICLH double cup] implant is Alan Swanson, who is sitting next to me.[32] I was the surgical half, and together we were at Imperial College. The reason it failed, apart from the fact that I, like many others, didn't know what we were doing surgically, was, as I now realize, that the polyethylene cup, articulating with a large head, as John Charnley said, was a particular risk. But in retrospect I think much more important was the fact that it was gamma-irradiated in air and thus although it started out as ultra-high molecular weight polyethylene [UHMWPE], by the time it was implanted into the patient, the chain lengths had usually been reduced and the wear rate went up through the roof. I don't know whether you want me to comment on cobalt–chrome-on-cobalt–chrome. I will do if you wish.

Another piece of Professor Swanson's work was the design – I don't know whether it was the first – of one of the earliest hip and knee simulators, in which he ran cobalt–chrome against cobalt–chrome and metal against polyethylene. In 1972 I put in my first resurfacing arthroplasty. A man called Trentani at the

---

[32] The ICLH double cup was implanted using a thin layer of PMMA in 1972, following two years of laboratory investigation. The prosthesis used on the first 16 hips had a HDP femoral component and a stainless-steel acetabular component. From 1974 the acetabular component was of HDP with a cobalt–chrome femoral component, as in Figure 18 and Appendix 3, page 106. Freeman *et al.* (1975); Freeman (1978b); Freeman *et al.* (1978).

Rizzoli Institute in Bologna had put one in a few months earlier.[33] About that time Alan [Swanson] was doing this work and we retained the debris from cobalt–chrome and that was implanted into rats. The results were published in the *Journal* [*Journal of Bone and Joint Surgery*].[34] The fact is that cobalt–chrome-on-cobalt–chrome is a perfectly satisfactory material mechanically, if properly manufactured. We now know how to do that. But whether it's going to be biologically satisfactory, is a completely open question, and since Alan's work with myself and a man called John Heath, on the implantation consequences of the debris,[35] there's been a lot of work to do with cobalt and chromium in the area of DNA and fertility, which is quite unknown to orthopaedic surgeons. So we await that with some interest.

Lettin: That leads very nicely on to what we are going to ask Professor Alan Swanson to speak about, but before we do that, is there anyone who wishes to make any comments about these implants, before we move away really from this very historical part?

Mr Kevin Hardinge: Just to mention that the cement was introduced by John Charnley to fix the Thompson prosthesis,[36] and he found that with his exposure it would reduce the movement of the stem by some 300-fold, so it was a parallel development.[37] When the double-cup PTFE failed, he then abandoned the

---

[33] Paltrinieri and Trentani (1971); Trentani and Olmi (1974); Trentani and Vaccarino (1978).

[34] Swanson *et al.* (1973).

[35] Freeman *et al.* (1969a and b).

[36] Thompson (1952). See Appendix 3, page 102.

[37] Mr John Older wrote: 'I am concerned about the precise detail of Charnley's use of cement both in the comments made by Hardinge and others. The history of acrylic cement began with its first synthesis in 1843, but it was not used in the human body until 1937, and then only as a denture base material. In the early 1950s Sven Kiaer of Copenhagen [Kiaer (1951)] and Edward Haboush of New York [Haboush (1953)] used self-curing methylmethacrylate in hip surgery. They used, as did Ken McKee in Norwich and Maurice Müller in Switzerland later, small amounts as a seating compound beneath the collar of the femoral prosthesis to allow it to settle over a perfect surface area. Very little cement was placed down the medullary canal. In the late 1950s, Charnley was looking for a substance he could use to support the cup and femoral prosthesis in bone. He went to see Dennis Smith, a lecturer in dental materials in charge of the material laboratory of the Turner Dental School, Manchester, who took some pink self-curing acrylic off the shelf and suggested he use it as a filler. Charnley's great contribution as a result of this visit was the formulation and elucidation of the principle of using large amounts of acrylic as a filler or grout. Charnley's observations led to his third monograph, *Acrylic Cement in Orthopaedic Surgery*, a classic on the subject.' Note on draft transcript, 10 July 2006. See Older (1986); Charnley (1970). See also note 9 and Appendix 3, page 102, which shows the Thompson prosthesis secured by cement.

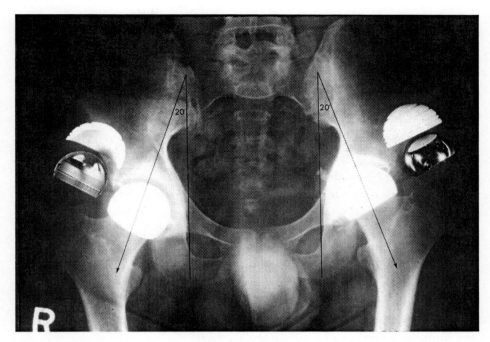

Figure 18: ICLH resurfacing arthroplasty done bilaterally, c. 1980.

plastic on the femur and switched to using a Thompson prosthesis with a PTFE cup and then he found that they were wearing out. The low-friction principle came about through serendipity, when he tried to increase the amount of plastic in the cup to extend the wear and he eventually ended up using a 7/8 inch stainless steel bar, which became the 22.225mm low-friction head. So the low-friction concept was found as a result of observation in trying to prolong the life of the implant.[38]

The other thing I would like to say is that John Charnley mentioned to me that he had done 300 of these hip replacements using PTFE, and they were all starting to fail and it was a very uncomfortable time for him. If he had been a surgeon working in the US, his back would have been nailed to the wall. Anyway, what he found was that the patients were still turning up at the clinic,

---

[38] Professor Mike Wroblewski wrote: 'Low-frictional torque was not a question of "serendipity"; it is a well known and accepted engineering principle. From the property of materials to low-frictional torque, the principle of the design was Charnley's application of mechanical factors to hip replacement. All this is well documented [Charnley (1961, 1974)]. Serendipity is certainly not the word to use in this context. Charnley did use the term in a broader sense.' Notes on draft transcript, 20 June and 24 October 2006. See note 27 and for an example of cup wear, see also Figure 5.

saying, 'We know the operation only lasts for three years, but we are having such bad pain, can you not do something?', because John Charnley's indication for a hip replacement was the patient's overall condition would be improved by a pseudoarthrosis, a Girdlestone operation.[39] So when they had all the implant material taken out, these patients were still better off than they had been pre-operatively. I think that should be recorded.

Miss Betty Lee:[40] It was a pleasure and a privilege to work for the late Mr G K (Ken) McKee. As a staff nurse and ward sister on the male orthopaedic block of the Norfolk and Norwich Hospital from 1950 to 1967, I observed Mr McKee's pioneering work on total hip replacement surgery, which he had commenced prior to 1950. He had frequent meetings with a Mr Hunton who owned a small engineering firm in Norwich. Together, they designed prototypes that surgical-instrument makers could then provide in the new inert metals. At that time, Mr McKee had treated arthritic hips surgically with lag-screw arthrodeses, whereas his colleagues, the late Mr H A Brittain and Mr R C Howard, favoured the V-type arthrodesis. However, in the early 1950s Mr Howard had treated two male patients suffering from ankylosing spondylitis with cup arthroplasties; later both the patients had total hip replacements.

Despite receiving little encouragement from the establishment, Mr McKee self-funded all his early research; official funding came only later. By the late 1950s a number of total hip replacements had been carried out successfully. After removing the head of the femur, a curved stem prosthesis was inserted into the medullary cavity above the trochanters, the cup being fixed into the acetabulum with a screw. Subsequently a new (metal) cup was used, with small projections on the outer side of the cup, which would fix into the dental cement then used to line the acetabulum. Mr McKee was very particular about the positioning of patients and relied upon the late Frank Baker, then theatre orderly (and, later, technician) to do this. In fact, he was reluctant to operate if Frank was unavailable. In the 1960s, Mr John Watson-Farrar joined Mr McKee as his registrar, later becoming the fourth consultant. Together they devised the McKee–Farrar hip joint. As a committed Christian, Mr McKee saw the alleviation of pain and suffering in others as his mission in life. It was to this end that he was a pioneer in total hip replacement surgery.

---

[39] See note 5.

[40] A memoir, prepared by Miss Lee in July 2006, 'Postwar development of the Orthopaedic Department of the Norfolk and Norwich Hospital', will be deposited, along with the tapes and other records of the meeting, in Archives and Manuscripts, Wellcome Library, London.

Freeman: This is a question to the group – is it true that there was a BOA meeting in Manchester or somewhere thereabouts, at a time when John [Charnley] was doing arthrodesis, and, so this story goes, Ken McKee came with some of his patients,[41] John [Charnley] saw the patients, and said, 'That's the way forward'; thus started replacement instead of arthrodesis. Is that true or is that rubbish?

Hardinge: The BOA meeting was in Manchester in 1960. I think the truth is that John Charnley was showing his cement fixation of the stem of a Thompson prosthesis in a fracture of the femur and that was the first time that Ken McKee had seen the use of cement in Manchester in 1960.[42]

Lettin: I can certainly remember Ken McKee showing his patients at the BOA meeting in Norwich when, in those days, we had a clinical meeting on Friday afternoon. He produced these elderly ladies with their dresses tucked in their knickers, and I think that was the last time there was ever a clinical meeting at the BOA. That was about 1963 or 1964.[43]

Kirkup: May I make a point about cement? We have forgotten Edward Haboush. I am talking about cement and total hips; in 1951, 1952, 1953, Haboush was using cement, methylmethacrylate. But, of course, he was applying it as a collar around the bone to support the prosthesis and this failed. The other point raised was 'who was doing total hips first?' I think McKee and Haboush are the significant pioneers, in the sense that they were using metal-to-metal and Haboush tried to use cement.[44]

---

[41] See McKee (1958).

[42] See Proceedings, BOA Spring Meeting, Manchester, 13–15 April 1961 [*Journal of Bone and Joint Surgery (B)* 43: 601; freely available online at www.jbjs.org.uk/archive/ (visited 8 November 2006)], where Charnley discussed his new form of low-friction hip arthroplasty and McKee reported that the failures of his similar operation involved loosening, but the use of cement was 'a great advance'. A clinical meeting was also held at the Manchester Royal Infirmary, with a clinical demonstration at Wrightington.

[43] Professor Mike Wroblewski wrote: 'The last clinical meeting of the BOA, unless there were later ones, took place 15–17 September 1982, the Manchester meeting. One session was in Wrightington Hospital with a presentation of a group of patients with the longest follow-up. Charnley died in August 1982. I presented the patients in September while Tristram Charnley did the filming. The record is available [Waugh (1990): 229–30].' Note on draft transcript, 20 June 2006. See also Proceedings and Reports, *Journal of Bone and Joint Surgery (B)* (1982) 65: 213 [freely available online at www.jbjs.org.uk/archive/], on the Autumn Meeting of the BOA at Manchester, with a memorial service for Sir John Charnley on 15 September 1982.

[44] Haboush (1953).

Craven: It went in the acetabulum. John Charnley used the cement and there was a hue and cry about it, people didn't want it. What is he using cement for? People didn't want this, and as Kevin [Hardinge] said the first time it was used at Wrightington, it was the [uncemented] Austin Moore prosthesis.[45] This chap came in, an 18-stone man, who had been to several consultants, they didn't know what was wrong with him, and I was in theatre with John Charnley when they did the operation. I don't know whether John Read was there or not, but when they opened him up the prosthesis was wagging about in the medullary canal, and that was the first time that John used the cement at Wrightington. And then when McKee started with his hip, where I say they were spiked, McKee got the cement through Charnley, and started cementing his sockets.

Lettin: I think we must move on, because we have touched on the materials and how the initial materials were not very good; we have talked about configuration; and Michael Freeman has also mentioned the biological side of it. I think it's time we brought in the engineers. Professor Alan Swanson, I would like you to talk about how the engineers became involved in this, and the importance of the materials, and the design and so on.

Professor Alan Swanson: I have been trying to think back 50 years, as no doubt other people have. Fifty years ago, I was employed, at a very junior level, in the making of aeroplanes in a laboratory in Bristol that dealt with materials, and one of the jobs I had was to write up the results of a long, continuing programme on the corrosion of so-called stainless steel. I can assure you that when you expose it to saltwater and air, it goes a lovely red colour.

The fact is, of course, that what is colloquially known as stainless steel is always corrosion-resisting steel on the specifications, not quite the same thing. However, back 50 or more years ago, what I shall nevertheless call stainless steel – iron with carbon and lots of chromium and nickel – had been around since 1913, and was well known for its corrosion-resisting properties: good for chemical apparatus, food handling apparatus and all that, and of course, implants, if only for fracture fixation. It was known to be very tricky stuff indeed if you tried to weld it, which was not normally a consideration. If, like Charnley, you had a solid head on the femoral prosthesis, you didn't think about making a hollow

---

[45] The Austin Moore metal hip prosthesis was introduced in 1940 as the first Vitallium prosthesis to replace the upper portion of the femur [Moore (1957)]. The most commonly used treatment of a displaced femoral neck fracture has been the uncemented hemi-arthroplasty and the cemented Thompson, although not entirely satisfactory. See Scales (1983); Weinrauch *et al.* (2006).

head and welding two bits together. It was also a bit dodgy in contact with itself. In general engineering, there was a prohibition on the use of stainless steel nuts against stainless steel bolts, for example. And therefore stainless steel for both components of a hip prosthesis is not, I think, something that any engineer would have recommended.

There were also cobalt–chromium-based alloys, which had been around in dentistry since the 1930s, and there had been some cross-fertilization or lateral thinking between orthopaedic surgeons and dentists, which had made people realize that they are on the whole at least as corrosion-resistant as the steel, perhaps more so, and somebody discovered, I know not who or where or when, that you could put cobalt–chromium alloys against themselves as a bearing pair without a disaster.[46] Titanium was more or less exotic. Going back to my days of making aeroplanes, I remember we were doing tests on titanium alloys for high-speed aeroplanes and it was fabulously expensive, fabulously difficult to do anything with, and therefore only of use in military applications, where in those days money was no object. That has changed, of course, and titanium alloys are now very respectable, although not good in general, as bearing materials.

If we turn to plastics, back in the late 1940s and early 1950s, there was nothing like the range of plastics we have now, and nothing like the understanding. Hence, polyethylene was polyethylene, and only later did the high-density and the high-molecular weight characteristics begin to be distinguished, and only later did we move on to UHMWPE with its extra wear resistance. PTFE was known then as a slippery plastic and one can understand why Charnley, or anybody else, might have thought it attractive as a bearing material against steel, although as we all know there were difficulties, and polyethylene, if the right kind, turned out to be better.

If we turn to ceramics, which I know were not in use then, but had been actually thought about and tried earlier, I think, for some interposition cups, way back, the point about ceramics is that you can make a much finer surface finish than with metals, which ought to lead to lower wear. Another good thing in their favour, if you are thinking of a bearing, is that unlike corrosion-resistant steels, which depend for their corrosion resistance on an oxide film that is likely to be rubbed off in a bearing and has to be continuously reformed (there are other troubles, as people here know, about the heads of screws in fixation plates), ceramics are the same stuff throughout, and so you don't have to worry about

---

[46] Confirmation from clinical experience is provided by Howie *et al.* (2005); Fisher *et al.* (2004).

the wear rate dramatically increasing because you rubbed off the protective surface film. They are also more wettable in general, by aqueous solutions, than metals, and, therefore, that commends them also as bearing materials. But of course, they are brittle, less so now than they used to be, because, as with the alloys and the polymers, over 50 years people have learned a great deal about how to make and process them. But they are still rather more brittle than most metals that would be used, and I therefore do have doubts about ceramic heads being put on a conical stub on a metallic femoral stem.

Lettin: We have another very eminent engineer here. Duncan Dowson, would you like to say something about the design? There are lots of variations of the shape of the stem and so on, and we perhaps should have mentioned, I suppose, Robin Ling's contribution. Unfortunately, Robin is unwell and couldn't be here, but we might mention it. It seems that there were lots of different designs of stem, but did it really matter?

Professor Duncan Dowson: It was interesting to hear Alan Swanson speak, because, like him, I was working in the aircraft industry before returning to the academic world. I had started some research on the wear characteristics of certain polymers, including polyethylene, for the defence industry, particularly for military aircraft. The industry required a bearing material that would operate in very strange environments, and particularly not be affected by the presence of water and high humidity.[47] I was doing that work early in the 1960s when I first met John Charnley. After his trauma with PTFE,[48] Charnley was seeking an alternative polymer and we have heard the fascinating story about how the ultra-high molecular weight polyethylene came to his attention. He must have heard, and I know not how, of the research contract that we had at that time with the Ministry of Defence, as he came over to Leeds to see some of the experimental work that we were doing. This was after he had started to use polyethylene, and he became fascinated with our tribological studies. One of my lasting impressions of John Charnley is that he was a jolly good engineer.[49] He wanted to understand the engineering and the physical principles by which these different combinations of material and different bearing configurations would work. Since that first contact, we had very frequent and stimulating exchange visits, myself to Wrightington and John to Leeds.

---

[47] Erli *et al.* (2003).

[48] Charnley (1966a).

[49] See, for example, Charnley (1965).

It is interesting that the word serendipity has been used about him selecting the 7/8 inch (22.225mm) diameter femoral head. When in subsequent years, I invited a colleague of mine, Michael Longfield, to do a mathematical analysis of this, he and John Charnley worked together and it was relatively easy to show that the optimum head diameter should be 50 per cent of that of the outside diameter of the cup, for maximum wear life, and that comes out, of course, at about 25–27mm.[50] Charnley's 22mm was fine, so whether we define that as serendipity or not, I don't know, but it was very close to the optimum diameter as far as wear life was concerned.

But wasn't that a question of manufacturing? [**From the floor:** Yes.] I think the diameter was convenient for standard material, but Charnley clearly presented his selection in terms of two sound biomechanics principles. He was rightly obsessed at the time with reducing the frictional torque and this can be achieved by (a) selecting acceptable materials with the lowest coefficient of friction and (b) by minimizing the torque arm or head diameter. McKee, I think, was a bit more interested at that time in the wear story, rather than the friction story, but John Charnley wanted to minimize friction, and minimize the frictional torque.

There are two ways that you can do that. One is to minimize the coefficient of friction between the sliding components, and PTFE was the polymer with the lowest known coefficient of friction, so he naturally used PTFE initially. But, secondly, in order to minimize the frictional torque, you need to use the smallest acceptable diameter, and he adopted 7/8 inch or 22.225mm. His biomechanics was jolly good. That was how I first came into contact with him, and since that time we have seen the story unfold and, as Alan Swanson mentioned, different and much improved materials, both for femoral heads and acetabular cups, have subsequently been introduced.

The ceramic story has also been fascinating. It is interesting that at the present time, the current range of toughened ceramics is extremely good. They are good as bearing materials, but also exhibit very little fracture potential. The metals are greatly improved and the manufacturing procedures are also improved. In the past we have talked very much about the alternative material combinations, such as metal-on-polymer, or indeed of metal-on-metal. Now there is a whole galaxy of possibilities, metal-on-metal, ceramic-on-ceramic, metal-on-ceramic,

---

[50] Charnley *et al.* (1969). Later work on wear includes Geller *et al.* (2006).

metal-on-polymers, ceramic-on-polymers and many of these are being very actively developed at the present time.[51] It would be interesting to meet again in another 50 years to see which comes through as being the best combination.

Lettin: We have talked a bit about wear and I think we rather neglected John Scales and the Stanmore THR. I think my recollections of the original Stanmore was that there was a cup that was fixed to the acetabulum with nails – we had a gun which fired these nails – and then another cup which actually slotted into that. I think from the wear point of view he [Scales] was very much involved. There was an engineer, Ian Duff-Barclay, who was seconded from British Petroleum and he designed, I think, the first total hip simulator. Charnley sent his prosthesis down to Stanmore to be tested. There was a whole row of these things working day and night, all around the room, chugging away, lubricated with bovine serum, to determine the wear properties of the joint components.

We ought to mention the custom-made prostheses and, I think, John Scales [Figure 19] was probably the first to develop custom-made prostheses, particularly with regard to the treatment of tumours. Of course, Ginger Wilson was very much involved with the treatment of tumours, as I was with the knee rather than the hip, but I think that his contribution to custom-made prostheses should be recorded.[52] Now it is very easy to do. I don't think Ron Ansell is here, is he? [No.][53]

Sweetnam: May I just say that you are absolutely right. I think that John Scales was the prime mover in this particular field, but we shouldn't forget that he did it in collaboration with Harold Jackson Burrows, the Bart's Consultant. I think the major step between Wiles' original concept of a total joint replacement and subsequent success was entirely due to two things: cement and new materials such as cobalt–chrome alloy and high-density polyethylene. It was the development of cement that later allowed the stem of the femoral component to be fixed within the medullary cavity of the femur. Wiles used stainless steel, which we have heard from Professor Swanson was doomed to failure; Wiles used no cement, usually bolting his prosthesis on the femur, which was doomed to failure. So I think it is those two factors – the new materials and the fixation

---

[51] Dowson (2001).

[52] Wilson (1953, 1971); Burrows *et al.* (1975); Bradish *et al.* (1987); Roberts *et al.* (1991).

[53] Mr Ron Ansell was unable to attend the meeting. He had been involved with the early development of the Stanmore artificial joint and was in charge of the design office at the Department of Biomedical Engineering, RNOH, Stanmore.

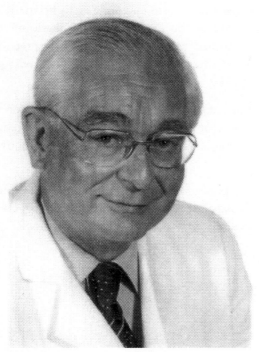

Figure 19: Professor John Scales, c. 1985.

by cement – that changed the whole spectrum of total joint replacement after Wiles' brilliant and original concept failed, because the suitable materials had not emerged in his day.[54]

Lettin: John Scales, of course, originally bolted in the prostheses and, I think, one of them replacing the distal femur and knee joint lasted for 18 years.

Mr Ian Stephen: I will speak on behalf of Robin Ling, who sends his apologies because he is unwell. I speak as a disciple of the originator, because I arrived in Exeter in 1976, about six years after the first Exeter prosthesis was implanted.[55] I think Robin's great contributions were: firstly, the stem geometry with the development of the double-tapered straight stem, and, secondly, the improved cementing technique that resulted in greatly improved fixation, as Rodney has been saying.

---

[54] Scales *et al.* (1965).

[55] The original Exeter Hip (EN58J) was available for use in clinical practice from autumn 1970. See Figure 20 and Appendix 3, page 105.

It is my recollection that we, as registrars, were encouraged to be meticulous about our cementing technique during the operation. The development of the straight stem double taper combined with improved cementing technique turned out, by serendipity, to have many advantages that were not envisaged at the time the Exeter hip was designed.

Lettin: Are there any more comments anyone would like to make on this? Malcolm Swann, did children present particular problems which required attention? I expect you had most experience dealing with children with juvenile rheumatoid arthritis.[56]

Mr Malcolm Swann: We were certainly very much in touch with Stanmore about children with juvenile chronic arthritis. I was persuaded by the late Barbara Ansell, who many of you will remember was a rheumatologist at the

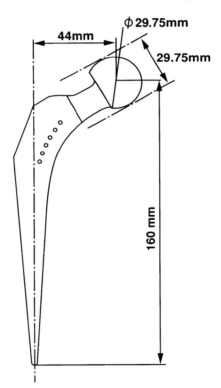

Figure 20: The Exeter stem, c. 1969.

---

[56] Ansell and Swann (1983).

MRC Centre for Rheumatic Diseases, Taplow, Maidenhead, who thought we should be able to help these children with their hip problems.[57] We are talking about children of 11 to 12 years of age and over, but they were all confined to wheelchairs with destroyed hips, and they could no longer manage the pain. We felt something should be done.

So we were faced with this problem of largely custom-made prostheses for them, because they had small skeletons. Children with juvenile arthritis are not just small, but they are smaller than small, they are minute. Graham Deane saw these as well. They have all sorts of problems, bone problems, hypervascularity, anatomical deviations, a lot of anteversion, so we did have to call on help from the custom-made prosthesis people. We did get a lot of help, particularly from Stanmore and John Scales. Of course, measuring at that time was very difficult, there was none of the technology of today, you merely had to take an X-ray with the artificial hip prosthesis held alongside the patient, judge that the magnification was roughly the same, and then send off the X-ray to Stanmore. Often we were held on tenterhooks, because there were a lot of telephone calls as to when it was going to be ready, and I can recall it was pretty well when the patient was on the table, a motorcyclist would arrive from Stanmore with the prosthesis in his pocket and you hoped that it would fit. Fortunately, mostly it did. I won't go into details of the numbers and so on.

Lettin: You mentioned manufacturers. Of course, the manufacturers were very important, and Phyllis Hampson is here. Well, Phyllis, I am not quite sure what your role with the manufacturers exactly was, with Zimmer Orthopaedic and, of course, as an intermediary with Stanmore. But I think we should also mention that John Charnley, of course, had an arrangement with Thackray's whereby they would not supply a Charnley replacement unless the surgeon had actually spent three days at Wrightington, in the tent, and learned how to do the operation. I in my time did exactly that, but I don't know how long that lasted, how long Thackray's kept that going.[58] Michael Wroblewski, you have got a comment on that?

Professor Michael Wroblewski: It was the second half of 1970. Sir John Charnley informed past Residents of the Centre for Hip Surgery at Wrightington Hospital

---

[57] Arden *et al.* (1970).

[58] Charles F Thackray Ltd of Leeds manufactured the Charnley prosthesis from 1963 until 1990 when Thackray's was acquired by DePuy, now a Johnson & Johnson subsidiary. See Foreman-Peck (1995): 109–10, 114. See also note 129 and Glossary, page 151–2.

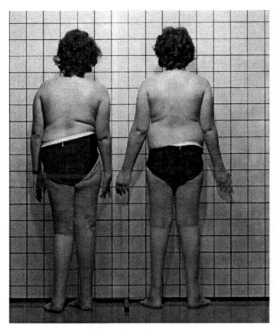

Figure 21: Still's disease – juvenile chronic arthritis – in plump male twins. The boy on the left has Still's, which shows in his posture.

by letter, saying that hip components generally were being made available under pressure from the manufacturers.[59]

Lettin: There you are, pressure from manufacturers. Phyllis, what about that? How much influence really did you have, or did the manufacturers have? You held the surgeons to ransom, I think?

Mrs Phyllis Hampson: No, I don't think that's true at all. I don't think we held the surgeons to ransom. We [Zimmer Orthopaedic] weren't really connected

---

[59] Professor Mike Wroblewski wrote: 'It was 1970: the facts are that the Charnley prosthesis was not patented. Charnley took no royalties: £1 sterling from the sale of each hip prosthesis was put into research. Charnley insisted on keeping the cost low, because "The NHS has to pay for it". The stem cost £18 and the cup £7. Other manufacturers were producing and copying the Charnley prosthesis. The manufacturer, Thackray, was constrained both by price and sales, hence the pressure from the manufacturer to make the Charnley prosthesis freely available.' Note on draft transcript, 20 June 2006. A history of Smith & Nephew suggests that the socket was sold for £3 and the femoral prosthesis for £12 in 1968, with Thackray paying £1 to the Wrightington research fund for every prosthesis sold. Thackray had sole manufacturing rights, while Wrightington retained control over quality. Foreman-Peck (1995): 109.

with any total joints until about 1970, when John Scales phoned us out of the blue one day, asking if we would be willing to make Stanmore total joints. My managing director at that time was Douglas Davidson, who would not, under any circumstances, make a total joint. But, luckily, just after that he went to Canada and the decision became mine. I decided that we were going into total joints with the Stanmore range. We started off having them made by Deloro Stellite, and then we set up our own company, Metallo Medical, in Swindon in 1970.

I don't think we held the surgeons to ransom, it was really John Scales who was holding us to ransom, because we had to promise not to make any other prostheses, apart from the Stanmore range, for at least two years, which we did and we kept to that. It went very well, and we started by manufacturing the metal-on-metal type [see Figure 17 on page 21]. I think we were the first company to make vacuum-cast implants, which meant that they were cleaner, hopefully, than making them air cast and the first one was inserted in 1963 by Ginger Wilson.[60] I believe the majority of metal-to-metal are still going very strongly. Prior to our own manufacture, the joints were made by Deloro Stellite and, I believe, Jackson Burrows was the first to insert one of these in 1956.[61]

Lettin: What about the British Standards for implants? Vic Wheble is here. Do you think that British Standards played an important part in this? How soon did they really come into having a standard?

Mr Victor Wheble: British Standards for clinical materials themselves started out as a technical committee in 1967 and this was chaired in the first place by Geoffrey Blundell Jones.[62] But by 1972 there was considerable interest from the Government, the Department of Health (DoH) and the corresponding Scottish organizations. So an international committee was set up and met in London at the British Standards Institution (BSI) headquarters. This was a special meeting called by Bernard Bloch of Australia, who suggested that perhaps this should be focused on international standards problems, and in fact there was no other committee existing at the time.[63] Bernard Bloch persuaded people from

---

[60] See note 29.

[61] Burrows (1966).

[62] For a detailed timeline of the British Standards Institution, see www.bsi-global.com/News/History/index. xalter (visited 12 July 2006). See also Appendix 2, pages 97–100, and Scales (1965).

[63] Bloch (1958).

various countries to come, and the first meeting took place in London, 27–28 March 1972.[64] This had representation from various other organizations such as the International Federation of Surgical Colleges and also from the various governments, of course, because they were interested in the fact that they were starting to supply prostheses for use in their hospitals. It went on from there. I only got into standards-making a little bit after that, because John Scales rang to ask me if I would join the committee, and I was on it from 1972 until 2004. I have actually had a lot of experience of all these committees.[65]

Now as far as distribution is concerned, I am only going to talk about John Scales' committee – he was chairman of the hip replacement committee – and he had many difficulties with the different people from all over the world, in arguing what could and couldn't be done. At meeting after meeting, these arguments occurred and eventually it got to the point where he threatened to resign. At that point, they decided that they had better just keep him, because he knew more about the whole subject than they did. Unfortunately, he was not able to be present at the 25th anniversary meeting of the ISO Technical Committee in Singapore in 1997, when he would have been awarded the special gold award from this committee, because of his 25 years of service.[66]

Lettin: I think you deserve a medal for staying on it for so long. It was the worst committee that I have ever been on, and I've been on a good many. I think you were representing the BOA and I was representing the College of Surgeons. Phyllis, you may remember – this is very pertinent to the Charnley cup. We spent a whole afternoon arguing the difference between a bevel and a chamfer. And I don't know what the answer was. John Paul – who was due to be here, but has had his knees replaced and couldn't walk all the way from Glasgow – tried to explain. It was a terrible meeting. 'Was the edge of the cup bevelled or was it chamfered'? This went on and on. Another question I can remember was: 'How far should the eye be from the end of a Küntscher nail'? I admire you, Vic, for staying on it for so many years.

---

[64] Bloch and Hastings (1972).

[65] See Appendix 2, pages 97–100.

[66] Mr Victor Wheble wrote: 'John Scales was a founder member of the ISO/TC150. I understand from Phyllis Hampson that John did receive his 25th anniversary award privately, later in 1997.' Note on draft transcript, 12 October 2006.

Wheble: May I just comment on the nail? That was a small group of rather old professors from France, backed up by other members from Germany, who could not agree that the hole at the end of a Küntscher nail had to be a certain size, not a whole series of sizes. Each country wanted its own particular size of hole in the nail, so that its own hook would fit. The argument continued until I managed to persuade them, after two hours sitting on a staircase in heated discussion with these eight people, that only one hole was needed, so if the largest hook would fit, so would the smallest!

Lettin: This BSI committee doesn't exist any more, does it?

Wheble: It does, it is still an active part of the BSI.

Lettin: What about the Medical Devices Agency? Didn't that take over from the BSI? [**From the floor:** No, it is not the same.] Oh, Keith, I didn't see you arrive, I am sorry about that. Would you like to say something about the Medical Devices Agency?

Mr Keith Tucker: The Medical Devices Agency (MDA) does not exist any more as it has been amalgamated into the Medicines and Healthcare Products Regulatory Agency (MHRA). You asked me to talk a little about regulations.

My introduction to orthopaedics was with Ken McKee and John Watson-Farrar in the late 1960s and so I learned about the things that you have been talking about today: ringing, polar bearing and so forth. I met Alan Chappell, a facio-maxillary surgeon in Norwich, who recommended putting the studs on the back of a McKee–Farrar cup. I remember those times very well and they were very informative years for me, given what I have been doing since then.

The prostheses in those days were matched, the socket and the stem came as a pair. This sometimes proved to be a problem during a revision. They [McKee and Watson-Farrar] were great people to work for and their prostheses did splendidly well. They were amazingly enthusiastic people, who commanded great admiration and sometimes bewilderment. Ken McKee's prayer session, at the beginning of each ward round, often in the middle of a large ward, was sometimes a daunting prospect to me as a young Senior House Officer. I took over McKee's firm as a Consultant in 1978 and it was in the 1980s when you [Lettin] seconded me from the Council of the BOA to the MDA. The MDA (now the MHRA) has developed considerably and perhaps you saw me as something of a poacher turned gamekeeper.

It was just before that time that a European Directive had come along (1994), which directed that all hip replacements would have to have a CE mark. As you know, CE markings are graded and hip replacements were type 3B.[67] Susanne Ludgate headed the MDA, ably assisted by Andy Crosbie and John Hopper. By 1998, all knee and hip replacements had to have the CE mark to conform with the European Directives. One thing that we immediately realized was that manufacturers could get a CE mark a year after the introduction of a new joint. Thus, provided the joints survived a year, they got their CE mark, and that, ladies and gentlemen, was how it was in 1998. There was no post-market surveillance and we were told that if we wanted to get into post-market surveillance we should have to turn over a European Directive from the European Commission, which sounded quite a formidable thing to do, even for orthopaedic surgeons. Realistically we got no further and, in fact, not as far as John Charnley. It is on record that John Charnley wanted to have some sort of joint registry right at the very beginning,[68] and it was, of course, at Charnley's instigation that surgeons could not acquire the tools to put in Charnley hip replacements without going to Wrightington to learn how.[69] It is also interesting to me that Ken McKee and John Watson-Farrar, although they started doing 'large volume' hip replacements in 1961, did not publish until they had five-year's data.[70] In their words, 'to see how they went'. Nowadays it is possible to put things in to the market more quickly.

---

[67] The letters CE are the abbreviation of the French phrase Conformité Européene or European Conformity. For details, see note 142.

[68] Sir John Charnley wrote in 1972: 'Serious consideration should be given to establishing a central registry to keep a finger on the pulse of total implant surgery on a nation-wide basis. Surgeons should not be permitted to perform total hip implant work (especially those involving the use of cement) unless prepared to have weekly returns made of the operations as they are performed, and thereafter to have patients questioned annually by circular from the registry'. Wrightington Hospial, Internal Publication no. 39, 1972 [see www.bitecic.com/events/Porter%20-%20What%20do%20Clinical%20Outcomes%20tell %20us.pdf (visited 9 November 2006)]. Jones (2000). The National Joint Registry for England and Wales was established in 2003 replacing the Trent and North West regional registers, and its first annual report, dated September 2004, is freely available from www.njrcentre.org.uk/documents/reports/part1.pdf (visited 17 July 2006).

[69] Professor Mike Wroblewski wrote: 'The Charnley hip replacement instruments were always freely available [to surgeons who had trained with Charnley]. To quote Sir John Charnley: "They could be used for other operations as well as hip replacement". This hip prosthesis was not available until the second half of 1970.' Note on draft transcript, 20 June 2006. See Figure 22.

[70] McKee and Watson-Farrar (1966).

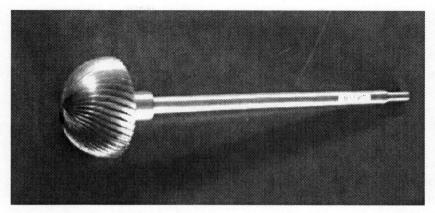

Figure 22: A Charnley acetabular reamer.

Lettin: Was that about the time of that BOA meeting in Norwich? Mike Freeman was asking me what year that was.[71]

Tucker: The BOA meeting in Norwich was in 1981, but the meeting you are referring to was actually at the Royal Society of Medicine in the 1960s.[72]

Lettin: I think we have covered quite a lot of ground. You were talking about registers and regulations and I think, Rodney and Mike, you were both quite keen on that, way back. I seem to remember that was another committee that I was on, but it came to nothing.

Sweetnam: You are absolutely right, it came to nothing. On your seats is a copy of a paper, the only paper that I have ever written that I think was of any value, and it concerns a scheme which our committee proposed. [**Lettin:** Was that a BOA committee?] No, it was a DoH committee called the Advisory Group on Orthopaedic Implants, and the report of that group is on your chair, dated May 1981.[73] I was chairman, Michael Freeman was a member, and after a lot of

---

[71] See note 43.

[72] McKee (1958). See also note 42.

[73] Sweetnam (1981). This report suggested a 'recommended list' of artificial joints considered by the Advisory Group to demonstrate adequate quality control during manufacture, the use of suitable materials, and of acceptable design. It was also mentioned in the recent review by Faulkner *et al.* (1998): 59–61, which noted the generally poor methodological quality of the 233 studies considered and that the results for different types of prostheses should be treated as estimates, although there were good results at ten years (given relatively poor evidence) for the Exeter, Lubinus IP, Charnley, Howse and Stanmore.

discussion, we came up with a scheme which would, I like to think, have spared us a lot of the disasters that have occurred in faulty joint replacements inserted thereafter. I repeat the date, 1981, a scheme put forward by our committee, accepted by the BOA, accepted by the DoH, indeed all the professional bodies accepted it. If it had gone into place, there would have been a surveillance scheme with a recommended list of prostheses, each prosthesis, each new design, would have been monitored. I repeat the date – 1981.[74] Accepted by the DoH and the whole profession, it never got off the ground.[75] My belief, and here I am going to come into conflict with another member in the audience, is that it never got off the ground because of the implant 'industry'. Now, Phyllis will tell me whether that is right or not, but I am told that someone in a senior position in the industry at that time, managed to persuade the DoH not to progress this scheme. And I would commend this paper to you, which was quite largely dependent on the work of Michael Freeman, I have to say.

Lettin: I thought he was the very important chap. Phyllis, are you going to respond to that barb?

Hampson: I really don't think it has anything to do with the trade at all, Sir Rodney. I think we had many problems. Let's be fair, Mr Ronald Furlong was never on any committee, not BSI, no BOA meetings, none of them.[76] I really don't think it was the trade who stopped the scheme.

---

[74] Professor Mike Wroblewski wrote: 'Charnley kept detailed records on punch cards. With the introduction of computers I had the information transferred to a very detailed database, which is updated after every visit and operation. This has formed the basis of the John Charnley Research Institute, a registered charity, with close to 30 000 records from November 1962 onwards.' Note on draft transcript, 20 June 2006.

[75] Mr Mike Heywood-Waddington wrote: 'I fully agree with Sir Rodney Sweetnam that it was a disaster, in terms of proper surveillance (see also page 39). The only local contribution I made was to ensure a regular follow-up of our own hip replacements (Charnley prosthesis through posterior approach), and ran a special hip clinic to achieve this, using the same methods of hip scoring and analysis as that used at Wrightington, for five years on an annual basis and then at five-year intervals. These results formed the basis of a successful thesis submitted for the MSc in Orthopaedics at the University of London by Mr S G Atrah FRCA in 1987, and were also the subject of a paper given by Mr John Dowell at the BOSG in 2003. A nation-wide register would, of course, have been far preferable.' Note on draft transcript, 11 October 2006.

[76] Sir Rodney Sweetnam wrote: 'Ronald Furlong was head of a very successful hip implant manufacturing company.' Note on draft transcript, 26 June 2006. Furlong's Joint Replacement Instrumentation (later JRI Ltd) became the sole licencee importing Müller components from 1971, later casting the components in titanium alloy in the UK at their Sheffield site. See details at www.jri-ltd.co.uk/ (visited 27 June 2006).

Freeman: It was a good scheme, everybody apparently agreed, but it did not appear. Historically, I would be very interested to know why not.[77]

Lettin: But wasn't it a question that it was limiting the implants that you and Rodney would have allowed? I seem to remember that the Stanmore knee would have been banned.[78] I think there was a perception that it would have been very restrictive.

Sweetnam: I am sorry, but it had the overwhelming support of the whole profession, including the BOA and there was no justification for not going ahead with it. The DoH agreed it, they asked me to write this paper, in a publication called *Health Trends*, which I did, quoting the DoH's acceptance. It did not get off the ground, and my understanding was that it was due to powerful voices within – I don't know whether they were members of the committee or not – the Surgical Trades Association.

Freeman: I think Rodney and I are both speculating that this was a scheme to which you could hardly object in public, so all the bodies said, 'Oh, well done', and then went out to the loo and said, 'Christ! As individuals we are not going to make any money if this comes off, so we must stop it.' But that is my guess [**From the floor:** Yes, I was in the loo at the time.].

Wroblewski: Mr Peter Frank, Consultant Orthopaedic Surgeon from Manchester, and I were approached by the DoH and we had several meetings on the subject. The object of the exercise was to have a Register, now incorrectly called a Registry, to put on record, first, all total hips, as well as hemi-arthroplasties. The project was obviously impossible for the two of us to do. I suggested that we could probably set up one locally, as a pilot scheme, to see whether this was going to be a working proposition. I suggested that to set it up from scratch would cost £250 000. That was the last time I heard from the DoH.[79]

---

[77] Sweetnam (1981). Sir Rodney Sweetnam wrote: 'The outcome was that there was no further action whatsoever, except that the DoH did introduce certain controls of materials and manufacture, which they called their Gold Standards, but never any clinical data or follow-up surveillance whatsoever. The DoH were simply too weak to grasp the nettle of "surveillance" and the only explanation I have for this is that they were not prepared to stand up to the "industry". All the medical professional bodies supported the scheme, but only the DoH had the power to introduce it.' Note on draft transcript, 7 October 2006.

[78] Mrs Phyllis Hampson wrote: 'I was never advised that the Stanmore knee should be banned. For what reason?' Note on draft transcript, 9 October 2006.

[79] Professor Mike Wroblewski wrote: 'My handwritten notes of the meeting are dated 7 July 1987'. Note on draft transcript, 24 October 2006.

Lettin: I think it has proved a very interesting discussion, which perhaps came a bit after the historical part, but nevertheless I think it is important that it has been reported. Kevin, you want to say a bit more?

Hardinge: For the historical record, when Stanmore started making their hip replacement, they did approach John Charnley to see if they would be able to market the Stanmore–Charnley; John Charnley wasn't too keen on this and he suggested that they should market the Stanley–Charnmore!

Wheble: There was an attempt at one time to do exactly that internationally, to get a standard where you could control some of these things, but it never came to anything at all. Of course, none of the companies was interested.

Lettin: It was difficult enough getting the standards through for the metal, wasn't it? Another thing that I can remember in that BSI committee was that the Swiss materials were very much worse than the British materials, the Americans somewhere in between, and we couldn't agree a standard. I think the Swiss were still using old railway lines. They had bought up the Burma railway and were manufacturing the prostheses out of old railway lines. We couldn't get an agreement: never mind an agreement on the design of prostheses, we couldn't get one on the materials that they were made from. It was a very boring committee. I think we have talked about regulation and it doesn't seem as though the manufacturers really hampered the orthopaedic surgeons, if Phyllis is to be believed. They didn't say, 'You can't make it like this'; they fitted in with whatever designs the surgeons produced.

Hampson: Sometimes one had a note on the back of an envelope, or a cigarette box, saying: 'Can you make this?' You had to go along with the surgeon up to a point, but usually some modification had to be made, with the surgeon's approval.

Lettin: Are there any other points on the design or the materials? Michael [Freeman] mentioned the terrible fright that happened when he put all this wear material into rats and every lump that appeared in a patient that had had a hip replacement was thought to be a tumour [see page 22]. But, Michael, is there any more you would like to say on that? Or Alan [Swanson], for that matter.

Freeman: I am sure everybody knows. Alan [Swanson] knew, because he wrote it in a book that we edited, and I have just whispered to ask him if he would care to repeat what he said in the book, and he says he can't remember writing it.[80] So I have to ask the audience. The point is if you gamma-irradiate in air, you cross-link the chains, which may be good mechanically, but in oxygen you also split the chains so that, strictly, the material is no longer UHMWPE. For a long period we gamma-irradiated in air, at a time when the atomic industry knew perfectly well what would happen, in principle, if you irradiated polymers in air. A lot of the wear problems that I think we hit in the middle period, after the period you are talking about, Chairman, were due to that. My question is: can the early Wrightington people tell us how the polyethylene cup was sterilized to begin with? Secondly, when gamma-irradiation was introduced, whether consideration was given to the downside mechanical consequences? I should say that I've whispered to John Read, and he says he can't remember, but maybe Mike Wroblewski or somebody else can. Why did we gamma-irradiate in air without knowing what we were doing?[81]

Wroblewski: Until March 1967, the cups were machine-washed, soaked in formaldehyde, washed again, and then implanted. From March 1967 onwards, the manufacture was transferred to Thackray's in Leeds, and it is at that stage that they were gamma-irradiated.

Tucker: Very briefly, following on from what Michael was saying, I think one of the important parts of the history, certainly as far as I am concerned, was in the mid-1970s, when Michael published his paper showing that allergy to metal ions,[82] or what was thought to be allergic reaction, which he alluded to before, I think, probably finished off the metal-to-metal argument, certainly for quite a while. Perhaps it was the early 1970s, Michael, when you showed the acetabular components on metal-to-metal prostheses going in to the pelvis.[83] If you can't remember, I can.

Freeman: I don't want to get into minutiae; I did publish on that subject, but I wasn't the first to publish on the issue of whether cobalt–chromium was in the hair, urine and so on.[84] That wasn't actually the point I was making, which was:

---

[80] Professor Alan Swanson wrote: 'Professor Freeman credits me with too much. In the book referred to [Swanson and Freeman (1977): 164] I mention the degradation of mechanical properties caused by irradiation, but not the difference between irradiation in air and *in vacuo*.' Note on draft transcript, 26 June 2006.

[81] Shen and Dumbleton (1974); Black (1978); Besong *et al.* (1998).

[82] Evans *et al.* (1974); Benson *et al.* (1975); Elves *et al.* (1975); Lalor *et al.* (1991).

[83] Heath *et al.* (1971).

[84] For example, Coleman *et al.* (1973).

why did we sterilize by gamma-irradiation in air? Was it that nobody knew any better? Why was it? I mean, looking back, it was an incredible thing to do.[85]

Mr Krishna (Ravi) Kunzru: A bit of an anecdote on a totally different subject: I was Malcolm Swann's and George Arden's senior registrar, and I remember George Arden trying to put one of those custom-made prostheses into a child and it just wouldn't fit. The reason simply was that the stem was too long and we had to get a carborundum disc to cut the stem off in the theatre. We had to find the engineer first – I think he had gone home. We lived through rather interesting times.

Lettin: I think Ian Stephen touched on the pressurization of cement, because that was something that probably came about in this period that we are talking about. Certainly, John Scales was pressurizing the massive implants in humans, and he had a gun, which he got from De Havilland – it's funny how the aircraft industry is mentioned again – which worked off an oxygen cylinder and it was really quite a fearsome thing and I had a certain amount of experience [with it] just after I got on the staff at Bart's.[86] It was a patient with a tumour of the upper end of the humerus and John might have been possibly one of the earliest, I don't know, to ream [scrape with a reamer, see Figure 22] the medullary cavity. He brought his own reamers with him, which I think he probably got from the ironmongers, and when he got to reaming the humerus I had exposed, he said: 'You had better let me do this, it's a bit tricky', and so he reamed the shaft of the humerus. Then it came to putting in the cement, and he said: 'You had better let me do this, this is a bit tricky', and my house surgeon, who was holding the arm then, said: 'Does it matter, sir, but the elbow's swelling?' John had obviously drilled through into the elbow joint and the cement was going into the joint. He said: 'What are we going to do now?' So I said: 'We'll put that prosthesis in as fast as we can'. We put the prosthesis in and then we took a plug of cement out from the elbow joint. John was in at the crack of dawn the next morning to see this patient, who had nothing worse than a transient ulnar nerve palsy [due to compression of the nerves].

---

[85] See note 81.

[86] Mr Michael Wilson wrote: 'As I remember the hammer/drill was one of Scales' inventions – a pneumatic, percussion hammer, which relied on ball bearings to provide the percussion element. I don't think it lasted beyond the Heath Robinson stage, as the ball bearings would periodically fall out all over the theatre floor and have to be retrieved.' E-mail to Mrs Lois Reynolds, 9 November 2006.

Mr Tristram Charnley: On the question of sterilization, I certainly remember in the early 1980s, and Mike Wroblewski can probably confirm this, but Thackray were vacuum-packing the cups before sterilization.

Freeman: I am very sorry, because Thackray's were doing it in the 1970s, or not until the early 1980s, somewhere there. So, can I ask Phyllis: why did the rest of industry go on gamma-irradiating in air?

Hampson: I am terribly sorry, I have no idea.[87]

Freeman: But they were vacuum-packed and then sterilized. So, they were sterilized in a vacuum. [**From the floor:** Well]. What do you mean 'well'? They were sterilized in a vacuum.

Ring: Mike Freeman has mentioned the possible toxicity of the metal-on-metal bearing and, I think, historically it's important to record this. For that, and perhaps for other reasons, Ken McKee turned to metal-on-plastic in or around 1980, and I did the same thing. Reports of toxicity, mostly if the implants were made out of cobalt, came from John Scales and from Mike Freeman, and the metal-on-plastic joints seemed to be giving rather better early results.[88] In spite of the possibility that metal ions are hazardous, one way or another, there has been a resurgence of metal-on-metal joints. Perhaps progress is circular.

Lettin: I think Professor Swanson made this point earlier: that it was a question of the purity in the manufacture of the metals, which is so much better now. Perhaps that connects up with the Swiss railway lines.[89] I think we should move on to the question of the operation. Each of the early pioneers seemed to adopt a different technique. Charnley, as we all know, took off the trochanter, which

---

[87] Mrs Phyllis Hampson wrote: 'When I left school I went to work at the London Splint Company, which was owned by an American, Mr F I Saemann. In 1947 he sold the company and decided to start a manufacturing unit [Zimmer Orthopaedic Ltd]. The place he eventually chose was in Bridgend, South Wales. In 1968 or thereabouts the Managing Director of the company decided to live in Canada, hence my promotion to MD. When Mr Saemann died, his heirs decided to sell the company to Biomet [now Biomet Merck]. I stayed with them for a short while and then decided to retire in 1985. Unfortunately when Biomet bought the company, they closed and dismantled the London office and the manufacturing unit in Swindon where the total joints were made. All of the history of the companies was destroyed.' Letter to Mrs Lois Reynolds, 26 June 2006. Mr Ravi Kunzru wrote: 'Zimmer bought the Swindon works from the firm Deloro Stellite, who had been making hip parts there for many years.' Note on draft transcript, 16 October 2006. See also pages 34–5.

[88] Coleman *et al.* (1973); Heath *et al.* (1971).

[89] See page 42.

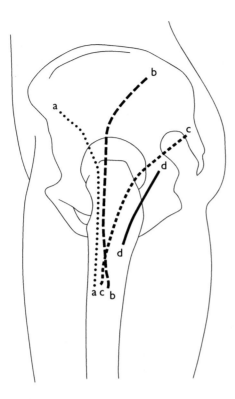

Figure 23: Surgical approaches used in total hip replacement.
L to R: (a) anterolateral incision; (b) direct lateral incision;
(c) lateral or posterior incision; and (d) modern minimally invasive incision.
Drawn by Mr Kevin Hardinge.

I think he tried to rationalize, but those of us in the south, perhaps, were more used to a posterior approach. Kevin [Hardinge], you developed an approach of your own.[90] But perhaps we should start off with Mike Waddington and Ken McKee's approach to the hip, which was an anterior approach [see the anterolateral incision in Figure 23], wasn't it? We have got some film later,[91] both of McKee and Charnley, but I think we will put those on during teatime so that people can have a look while they are drinking a cup of tea.

---

[90] Hardinge (1982). For a more recent evaluation, see Barrack and Butler (2005).

[91] The 1966 film of Ken McKee operating, digitized on DVD, and a digital copy of the silent film of John Charnley's operation will be deposited, along with the tapes and other records of the meeting, in Archives and Manuscripts, Wellcome Library, London.

Mr Mike Heywood-Waddington: Reference has been made to serendipity, and I have to admit that my professional career was largely based on serendipity, rather than on any structural planning. One of the best examples of that is really how I got to meet Ken McKee. While working as senior registrar for the late Herbert Seddon at the RNOH, I was summoned to his office, which, as you remember, Chairman, was slightly preferable to being invited to his rose garden.[92] He said that he wished me to go to Norwich to act as the late Ian Taylor's locum there, while he carried out a stint at Kano, Nigeria.[93] As a result I spent four months at the Norfolk and Norwich Hospital from September 1965 to January 1966.

There was another item on the agenda, because, as I think you may testify, there was some scepticism amongst the staff at the Royal National Orthopaedic Hospital (RNOH) at Stanmore about the real merits of what was going on both in Wrightington and in Norwich, from Jackson Burrows in particular. So my instructions were to report back on the McKee hip: 'Waddington, get this very clear, does the Norwich hip work, and will it last?'

Anyway, I went up there and everybody at Norwich was extremely kind to me, nobody more so than Ian Taylor, with whom I stayed before he departed for Nigeria. John Watson-Farrar and Ken McKee took me through the operation. I explained that I was being pressed to report back to the RNOH and asked if I could make the film [shown during the meeting's tea break],[94] because I felt that if I couldn't show McKee himself performing the operation, it might be thought that I was introducing my own modifications when I returned to Stanmore.

---

[92] Mr Michael Wilson wrote: 'Concerning Sir Herbert Seddon's rose garden, my father ['Ginger' Wilson] wrote the following for his speech to the Seddon Centenary, which would have been around July 2003: "The mere mention of a visit to the Rose Garden was sufficient to put the fear of God into any registrar in training; for they knew it could be a prelude to being gently moved on. As a consultant I was never summoned there; for as I have already explained HJS [Sir Herbert Seddon] had other methods of dealing with recalcitrant junior colleagues. But JTS [John Scales] seems to have been a fairly regular attender. His experiences are worth recording, and I quote: "As we progessed through the garden engaged in erudite discussion, every now and then HJS would stop, bend forward, pick a weed from the lawn, and then continue his point. This method of progression could be somewhat disconcerting to a nervous visitor".' E-mail to Mrs Lois Reynolds, 17 October 2006.

[93] Mr Alan Lettin wrote: 'HJS asked me as his First Assistant to find locums for consultants going to Kano.' Note on draft transcript, 25 November 2006.

[94] See note 91.

But you are quite right, I should add that I was very privileged to know Ken McKee very well for a long time: he used to come down and stay with us when he operated from time to time at the Essex Nuffield Hospital, Brentwood, after his retirement from the NHS. I also went on a regular basis to the well-known annual meetings of the British Orthopaedic Study Group (BOSG) at Zurs, Austria, attended by both McKee and Charnley.[95] There was a lot of free and informal discussion through the 1970s from both of them, from which I learnt a lot.

You are quite right that both Charnley and McKee had an almost doctrinal attitude to their surgical approach: McKee's was the anterolateral approach (the Watson-Jones approach),[96] and, of course, Charnley insisted on a lateral approach with trochanteric osteotomy. Charnley told me later that Kevin Hardinge would be allowed to do things his way, if he [Charnley] needed the operation himself.[97] However, the film shows the operation as performed by McKee, so I think it can speak for itself.

Lettin: The great problem with that approach was the chap under the sheets [the technician who manipulated the leg as required by the surgeon], wasn't it?

Heywood-Waddington: Yes, and as you know we had our Terry [a technician] and, I think, they had their Keith [a technician] – I can't remember his name – at Norwich. I have to say that that part of the technique was one thing that I gave up when I got my own consultant's job, and adopted the posterior approach, for which I make no apologies.

Lettin: Mike [Wroblewski], did you continue to remove the greater trochanter throughout your working life?

---

[95] Mr Mike Heywood-Waddington wrote: 'Much of the conversation at the British Orthopaedic Study Group meetings was informal, but there exist minutes of the scientific papers given, which included regular contribution through the 1970s from both McKee and Charnley on their evolving views on the development of the artificial hip joint, and related matters. The proceedings are published annually, but have a private circulation to members, but can be made available to anyone properly interested who approaches the secretary, at present Mr Tim Morley. Their scientific validity is undoubted.' Note on draft transcript, 11 October 2006.

[96] The anterior surgical approach to the total hip replacement is one of the oldest, developed in the 1930s by Boston surgeon Marius Smith-Petersen, later modified by British surgeon Sir Reginald Watson-Jones, both of whom used this approach to repair fractures of the femoral neck. See Smith-Petersen (1930); Watson-Jones (1935); Charnley (1950b). See anterolateral incision illustrated in Figure 23.

[97] Jolles and Bogoch (2004).

Wroblewski: Mr Chairman, may I correct you. It is not merely a question of the trochanteric osteotomy, if we read Charnley's description of the method of exposure, it was quite purposeful;[98] all to do with the mechanics of the hip joint. To medialize the cup, reducing the medial lever while increasing the lateral lever by moving the trochanter laterally. We now have evidence to support that: medialized cups wear less, cups supported on the rim wear more.[99] It is not merely the question of exposure. In fact, in later years, Sir John Charnley used to say that he did not charge his private patients to do a hip replacement, he charged them for reattaching the trochanter [Laughter], clearly emphasizing the benefit of the reconfiguring of the hip joint mechanics.

The answer to your original question is yes – until 18 months ago when I retired from clinical practice.

Lettin: You have learned better since.

Wroblewski: That's a matter of opinion.

Lettin: The perception in the south was that this was the way that the Manchester surgeons approached the hip: that Sir Harry Platt did it this way, and his pupil John Charnley did it this way. Of course, surgeons in the south didn't approach the hip by taking off the trochanter, and that what you said was really an effort to rationalize the approach, which was the Manchester way. Now, we have some engineers here and I wonder whether they would go along with the thesis that Mike Wroblewski has put forward?

Mr Graham Deane: I am only half engineer [has an engineering qualification], but what came to mind is a recollection of another great man, Edgar Somerville, whose registrar I was in 1969. I remember when we were doing Charnley hip replacements, Edgar Somerville was in conflict with many of his colleagues because he would not take off the trochanter. I remember we were having a problem with a hip replacement, and Edgar Somerville said, 'I had better phone my friend John to see what's wrong'. He phoned John Charnley and, of course, you only hear one side of the conversation. He would be holding the X-ray in

---

[98] Charnley and Ferreira (1964). Charnley's technique for transplantation of the greater trochanter is represented there in Figures 3–8.

[99] Wroblewski *et al.* [(2004): 499, Table 2] suggest that the medialized cup position contributed to both the low and high wear groups with a *p* value of 0.07. See also, for example, Perka *et al.* (2004).

his hand and he would describe it all, then came the obvious pause, and quite clearly the question that came back from John Charnley was, 'Did you take the trochanter off?', and Edgar Somerville would reply, 'Of course not, I never take the trochanter off'. The end of the conversation was always, 'You know why you are having a problem then'.[100]

Lettin: But that was a question of his approach, not the mechanical notion, which I was hoping the engineers might have.

Deane: The mechanical notion is certainly true, the practicalities of it were different. Another recollection of mine was from a visit to Wrightington. One thing that always puzzled me was that the laboratory, which had all the various test rigs, there were more test rigs on how to reattach the greater trochanter than for anything else. That always concerned me. Everything else was a single technique, but, from a practical point of view, the trochanter was obviously causing quite a bit of trouble.[101]

Lettin: That reminds me of a BOA meeting when John Charnley was reading a paper, I think, on his latest technique for fixing the greater trochanter back,[102] which I am sure Mike Wroblewski must admit did sometimes prove to be difficult, and a senior registrar by the name of Chris Colton got up and was

---

[100] See note 103. Professor Mike Wroblewski wrote: 'The history of trochanteric osteotomy in THA is well documented [Wroblewski (1990): 19–28]'. Note on draft transcript, 20 June 2006.

[101] Professor Mike Wroblewski wrote: 'Visitors to Sir John Charnley: Michael Freeman (6 May 1965); Alan Swanson (6 May 1965); Ken McKee (26 August 1966); Alan Lettin (April 1967); John Scales (15 May 1969); "Ginger" Wilson (15 May 1969). Sir Robert Jones, Liverpool, visited Wrightington Hospital on 2 October 1932.' Note on draft transcript, 20 June 2006. A copy of a page from 1932 of the Wrightington Hospital's visitors' register will be deposited along with other records of this meeting in Archives and Manuscripts, Wellcome Library, London. Mr Mike Wilson wrote: 'I've checked my father's diary for May 1969 when he went up to Wrightington. I enclose the following extracts: "14th May 1969: Went up to visit John Charnley today driven by John Scales [John was notorious for his driving technique]! Just after doing 92mph down a hill we had a flat tyre!" "15th May 1969: Usual six arthroplasties in the day. A few more new gimmicks. He [John Charnley] has a good way of bringing the fat together with tension sutures and sponge protectors for the skin and a very neat way of using the stockinette as a dressing".' E-mail to Mrs Lois Reynolds, 17 October 2006.

[102] See note 98. For details of the different approaches to the trochanter, see links from www.wheelessonline.com/ortho/modified_hardinge_anterolateral_approach_to_the_hip (visited 27 July 2006).

greeted in absolute silence when he said, 'Why do you want to make an easy operation difficult?' There was absolute silence.[103]

Sweetnam: The last few contributions, I think, are pretty fundamental. What is this business of removing the greater trochanter? I went to see Sir John operate and I came back to London and I did his operation and I always took the greater trochanter off. I went to great pains to put the greater trochanter back exactly where it had come from, because that is what I thought I had been taught. Now I have seen specimens from, I think, his test rig, testing the methods of fixation, and it looks to me as though it was done in the way I did it, that the greater trochanter was put on exactly from where it came. Now we hear that it's fundamental that the greater trochanter is put somewhere else. I would like to have this sorted out. I believe there is a myth out there about any significant shift in its position.[104]

Lettin: Alan Swanson is going to sort it out for you.

Swanson: I will say nothing about the problems of reattaching the greater trochanter, but I must say, as an engineer, I was most impressed when I read and re-read Charnley's account of the operation, because it did seem to me that he was designing a process of which the prosthesis was part, and the idea of accepting that the centre of gravity of the body is where it is, moving the centre of the hip joint closer to that, to decrease that medial moment arm, and increasing the lateral moment arm of the abductor muscles, by moving the greater trochanter laterally, where you reattach it, thereby reducing the total level of force on the hip joint.[105] It made excellent mechanical sense. Whether it makes better sense surgically or not I am not competent to say, but I was

---

[103] Professor Christopher Colton wrote: 'I recall that at a BOA meeting at the Royal Festival Hall – can't recall the year – there was a paper by Charnley on trochanteric osteotomy fixation. I recall commenting that all these methods of fixation were fine and dandy, but that it was not necessary to take off the greater trochanter in the first place. I think I complimented him on finding an elegant solution for a problem of his own creation. That went down like a pork chop at a bar-mitzvah – no wonder my career almost sank without trace. I do recall Michael Freeman agreeing with me publicly.' E-mail to Mrs Lois Reynolds, 2 October 2006. The BOA meeting at the Royal Festival Hall was held 13–18 September 1976. E-mail from David Adams, Chief Executive, BOA, 2 October 2006. See Proceedings and Reports [*Journal of Bone and Joint Surgery* (February 1977): 59] freely available at www.jbjs.org.uk/cgi/issue_pdf/frontmatter_pdf/59-B/1.pdf (visited 9 November 2006).

[104] Charnley and Ferreira (1964). See discussion on page 49.

[105] Charnley (1961, 1979).

impressed by what, I suppose, these days would be called holistic thinking, rather than, 'Let's just design a prosthesis'.

Lettin: That's very interesting. Duncan Dowson, you had been going to say much the same, I think. You were shaking your head in the affirmative.

Dowson: Yes, I cannot make any comments on the surgical aspects of this, but I agree with Alan and I have enjoyed the last few minutes of the discussion.

Freeman: Can I slightly endorse Rodney's point and read into the record the fact that I think that the first person to do Charnley's operation outside Wrightington, was John Read at the London [Hospital]. I am not sure if that's true, I wonder if anyone can improve on that recollection of mine. And then to just make a brief contribution to the 'where do you put things' issue, I quite see Alan's point that it's a process, and it's a rational process, but I must say as a surgeon, I fear I had the same problems as Rodney, that I couldn't actually put the trochanter anywhere else, even if I had wanted to, and the idea of medializing it a lot has occasionally led to the odd problem that I seem to have seen, because you have only got a millimetre or two that you can reasonably go, haven't you?

Wroblewski: Sorry to take up so much time. I refer those unbelievers to the Swedish Hip Register to have a look for themselves at the results according to the exposure.[106] But the thing that fascinates me is that discussions often end up on the opinions of trochanteric osteotomy. I have never, ever heard anybody who advocates trochanteric osteotomy arguing against another exposure. I get the feeling that those who didn't have the proper exposure, somehow feel guilty that they are missing something. Am I correct?

Mr John Older: I just speak as one surgeon from the south of England who does the classical Charnley low-friction arthroplasty with a trochanteric osteotomy. And with my four and a half years working as an assistant and colleague with Sir John and following his very accurate and detailed explanation to me of his theory, I very much support what was said by our two engineers, Swanson

---

[106] Located at the Sahlgrenska University Hospital, Sahlgrenska, Göteborg, the Swedish nationwide study has been collecting and analysing data provided on a voluntary basis on all primary total hip replacements and revisions performed since 1979. Professor Peter Herberts and Associate Professor Henrik Malchau direct the study, supervised by a board elected by the Swedish Orthopaedic Association. See Malchau (1996). For further details, see www.jru.orthop.gu.se/ (visited 7 June 2006). The British debate favouring a national hip registry suggested that, over time, the Swedish registry reduced the range of different prostheses implanted, resulting in lower revision rates and improved surgical technique. Jones (2000).

and Dowson, together with Wroblewski. I was very impressed with Charnley's engineering arguments. The trochanteric osteotomy I have done throughout my career and never had any major problems – well, everybody has the occasional problem – but I found it successful and you do need it. Replying to Sir Rodney, it is correct that you don't put the trochanter back exactly where you got it from, that's part of Charnley's concept.

Lettin: I suppose at the end of the day there is little difference between the patients who have had their trochanters removed and stuck back lower down, and those who have not? I would be very surprised if there was any clinical evidence that the functional result was any better. Does anybody know?

Stephen: It is my recollection, and indeed in his history of the Exeter hip, Robin Ling has written that he considered the offset of the stem to be very important.[107] The original 44mm offset was to increase the abductor power by increasing the lever arm; this is another way of achieving the same effect. Another part of the rationale in the design of the Exeter hip was that it was specifically to be implanted through the posterior approach, which was commonly used in the south of England at the time [see Figure 23.].

Hardinge: I introduced the direct lateral approach, because I had seen a lot of problems with the Tobin trochanteric osteotomy, even if you have been trying to restore it in the proper position, it would fragment – the bone was diseased or whatever – or the wires would fracture. The thing I think people are missing is that you need to restore Shenton's line.[108] Movement of the trochanter distally, or moving it laterally, or getting supposed improved leverage by re-placement of the trochanter in some exotic position is a myth. The fundamental aim is to restore Shenton's line, that's what you do.

Lettin: Is Wroblewski going to speak to you after this?

Hardinge: I don't know, you just have to have quite an open view. The anterior approach, the Watson-Jones approach, I look upon as the cat burglar's approach to the hip. The posterior approach I look upon as the trademan's entrance to the hip joint. You must have the patient lying in the supine position to be able to place the implants correctly. So you need trochanteric osteotomy, if

---

[107] Ling (1997): 9–11.

[108] See Glossary, page 152.

there's an anatomical deformity around the hip.[109] I will be the first to say that you must use a trochanteric osteotomy if there's some abnormality in this case, but if this was a perfectly straightforward anatomical case, then why take the trochanter off?

Lettin: I think that was the point that Chris Colton was making all those years ago.[110] Keith, what approach do you use? I ought to know because you recently replaced my hip.

Tucker: Yes, you should! I continue using Ken McKee's approach with some modifications. Ken always thought that the anterolateral approach would cause fewer dislocations.

Lettin: But it's not Kevin Hardinge's approach?

Tucker: Alan, when did the long posterior lip come in from Wrightington? Because I think that's part of the history.

Lettin: I can't answer that. What about Mike Wroblewski?

Wroblewski: The long posterior wall Charnley cup was introduced in 1972. It was brought in to pacify some US orthopaedic surgeons who were worried about the dislocation of the hip. In fact, for the record, if I may, looking at 22 066 primary LFAs over the past 32 years, there were only 55 revisions for dislocation (0.25 per cent).

Tucker: Alan, if I could just go back to the question about dislocation, which we haven't discussed in a big way. Dislocation has been part of the history of hip replacement and formed a lot of the discussion in the last 25 years. It has been perceived that the posterior approach is the one with the greater dislocation rate, compared with the anterolateral approach.[111]

Lettin: We intend to have, as far as I can make it happen, a section after tea on complications and dislocation would be one of them, but there's no reason why we can't pursue that particular topic now. For the record, we have got the reason for people adopting different approaches. Kevin has explained quite clearly why he thinks his approach is satisfactory. Mike Wroblewski has focused on the well-known Charnley approach and it's very interesting that the engineers have

---

[109] See Glossary, page 153. See also Figure 23, page 46.

[110] See note 103.

[111] Higuchi *et al.* (2003).

actually said, 'This is sensible', although I think the experience of some surgeons is that it makes an easy operation difficult. But it's interesting that we have got it for the records, because there was a considerable debate early on. I don't know whether we have any current surgeons here, everybody is retired, except Keith [Tucker], who is the only one here still doing joint replacements.

The more precise details of the approaches,[112] perhaps it's my fault that we put back the showing of the film, because I thought that you would all have a lot more to say, but you have all been terribly good and nobody has spoken for more than four minutes, and not everybody has spoken. Before we go to tea are there any other people who want to come into the discussion, on any of the aspects?

Mr Geoff King: I was quite unsure why I was invited to this meeting, to be among the orthopaedic great and good of the country, and it now occurs to me that I am something of a living fossil. In 1963 I had a road traffic accident and was admitted to the Norfolk and Norwich Hospital under Ken McKee and, at the time, John Watson-Farrar was his senior registrar. He put a Küntscher nail[113] in my left femur, which I still have. Some five years later, I was working as a technician in the orthopaedic theatre with Ken McKee and John Watson-Farrar.

There are two things that I can recall, one may be slightly apocryphal about the design of the McKee hip. He didn't just turn to engineering, he also turned to tenth- and eleventh-century architecture. He copied the flying buttresses of Norwich Cathedral for the shape of the stem of his prosthesis [see Figure 6, page 9].[114] I was also a 'Frank' at one stage, in that I was under the covers manipulating the hip. During part of my career, I also remember that Watson-Farrar had a unique operating facility, in that he had very strange little fingers, with which he could poke the cement down the femoral stem.

To continue my timeline as a bit of an antique, I actually had a hip replacement in May [2005], through the posterior approach, despite the fact it was done in Norwich. I think it was the Birmingham resurfacing, nothing too serious.[115]

---

[112] A digital copy of the silent film shown on 14 March 2006 will be deposited, along with the other records of the meeting, in Archives and Manuscripts, Wellcome Library, London.

[113] A Küntscher nail, or intramedullary rod, was in frequent use until the 1970s and is a hollow rod of varying lengths and diameters secured to the medulla. See Glossary, pages 149–50.

[114] Professor Mike Wroblewski wrote: 'The flying buttress was the basis of extra-articular (Norwich) hip arthrodesis [Brittain (1941, 1942, 1948); Langston (1947)].' Note on draft transcript, 20 June 2006.

[115] See Appendix 3, page 106

Lettin: I did ask Mike Freeman why his double cup wasn't awfully well received, whereas McMinn's seemed to be. I hear McMinn sold his firm for £60 million, I don't know whether that's true or not.[116]

Freeman: Yes, I am afraid I didn't sell anything for £60 million, but there you are. The operation of resurfacing with polyethylene failed in everybody's hands, I think, including dramatically in my own, and, I think, that was mainly because of the production of polyethylene debris, plus a level of surgical experience, which wasn't what it is now.[117] The polyethylene debris I think was partly due to the size of the head – a point that Charnley made to me, and he was absolutely right – but, I suspect, overwhelmingly, that the polyethylene was not UHMWPE, because it had been sterilized by gamma-irradiation in air, and that this was the significant fact.

Derek McMinn's operation is plainly a success, and it has the great attraction that a cobalt–chrome acetabulum is thinner, so you get more space for the two components.[118] The engineering, as Alan has said, has improved, so the thing works from a mechanical point of view. I have to say that I don't think we know what the long-term effects will be in younger people, of persistently elevated cobalt and chrome levels in the blood. It is now known that those ions, of all the transitional metals, are DNA splitters, which they share with X-rays, and if you talk to the fertility doctors, they are a little bit concerned about it, so we are going down into an age group where this is potentially a problem.[119] Whether it will be, goodness only knows. But I think that answers your question, Chairman, doesn't it?

Lettin: I think so. It reminds me of a question that I was going to put earlier, about patenting these devices. I think, Lady Charnley, that John never patented the original hip joint [No], but he did subsequently [Yes]. And what about Ken McKee? Does anybody know whether he did?

---

[116] Midland Medical Technologies Ltd now trades as Smith & Nephew Bromsgrove Ltd.

[117] Freeman *et al.* (1975); Cameron and Freeman (1977); Freeman and Brown (1978); Freeman (1978a) [Issue 134 of *Clinical Orthopaedics and Related Research* contains articles by all the surgeons who had developed resurfacing arthroplasties.]; Freeman *et al.* (1978); Freeman and Bradley (1982); Levack *et al.* (1986); Hernandez-Vaquero (1987); Cotella *et al.* (1990).

[118] McMinn *et al.* (1996). See also McMinn and Daniel (2006); Daniel *et al.* (2006); McMinn *et al.* (2005); McMinn (2003); Grigoris *et al.* (1993); Roberts *et al.* (1992).

[119] Cobb and Schmalzreid (2006).

Heywood-Waddington: Just a couple of points there. I don't think he ever patented it, that I am aware of. But he did make several things clear to me during the 1970s at a meeting of the BOA, I think in Oxford.[120] One point about metal sensitivity, he did not accept that that was a problem. I don't mean in the longer term that Mike Freeman was referring to, I don't think he directly commented on that, but as far as actual metal sensitivity, cobalt and chrome sensitivity, he dismissed this as a problem. The other thing that I think is important to say is that his paper in 1966, the definitive paper,[121] paid tribute to John Charnley for the introduction of methylmethacrylate, and also to John Scales for advising McKee that chrome–cobalt was the ideal metal to be used.

Professor Sir Christopher Booth: I am a complete outsider, but listening to this discussion as a historian of the twentieth century, one has to wonder whether you are giving the impression that this was all happening in an international vacuum. What is extraordinary about medical equipment and prostheses and so on, is that the US manufacturers almost always moved in on anybody's invention, took them over and then the US manufacturers become the people that did it. Is that what happened here? Or was it preserved in England?

Lettin: I think I might be able to throw some light on this because the cement – at least I think that Simplex C was the original bone cement – was manufactured in a back street in Stamford Hill in London and the owner of the firm was an American who happened to be a patient of mine, which is how I know the story, soon after I got on the staff at Bart's.[122] And there are people here who will know much more about the composition, but there were inhibitors in the compounds that had to be mixed together, and this company, North Hill Plastics it was called, had the patent on these inhibitors, and the US FDA (United States Food and Drug Administration) would not grant permission for the cement to be used.[123] So, the Americans fell quite behind, and the patients were coming over to this country for hip replacements. (Jill Charnley is shaking her head.)

---

[120] Mr Mike Heywood-Waddington wrote: 'It was a BOA meeting which I think was in Oxford at which the question of late (possibly neoplastic) effects of polyethylene debris was discussed.' Note on draft transcript, 22 June 2006.

[121] McKee and Watson-Farrar (1966).

[122] Phillips *et al.* (1971).

[123] In 1966 North Hill Plastics were located at 49 Grayling Road, London N16 [McKee and Watson-Farrar (1966)]. See Phillips *et al.* (1971), for discussion of its cardiovascular effects. For the properties of acrylic bone cement, see note 9.

This irritated the Americans no end, and I think the first person actually to do a total hip replacement in the US was Harlan Amstutz who had worked for a year at the RNOH [Stanmore] and went back to special surgery in New York with a McKee prosthesis in his pocket along with some cement and the FDA gave him permission to do a one-off operation in 1962/3. In the end, of course, the Americans bought out this company, but the owner knew that if he gave the formula to the US FDA it would be leaked and he could not afford to defend his patent against the big American companies.

Hardinge: The surgeons who had been to Britain to train, like Harlan Amstutz and Joe Dupont, went back to the US and they had a licence to use the cement on a limited basis. Joe Dupont, who worked at Wrightington, went back to Phoenix, Arizona, and had 300 patients under treatment, pre-operative assessment, operated, and in rehabilitation. He was in the big time. He had an overdraft when he went back to Phoenix, and later he sent a Christmas card to a chap he knew, Walter George, also from Phoenix, which said, 'Come quickly, Walter, the end is not in sight.' So this was answering the American dream.

Talking about patents, the other thing that happened in 1970 was that the firm Charles Bechtol discovered that the Charnley implant was not patented, so that's when they brought out the Charnley type, so it was available to US orthopaedic surgeons in their technical stand.[124] That's when John Charnley realized he could no longer control it. He had been very proper and tried to control it. So after that, it was thrown open and you could get the instruments and start operating.

Lettin: Could you say anything about the manufacturers' point of view, Phyllis, because I suppose they didn't want to manufacture stuff that was going to be copied.

Hampson: That's quite right, too. John Scales had all the Stanmore implants patented by the National Research Development Corporation (NRDC), and anybody who wanted to make Stanmore prostheses had to go to John Scales at RNOH, Stanmore, and nobody else made them until the licences lapsed. By this time our company had been sold to Biomet.[125] Zimmer Orthopaedic used to pay royalties to the NRDC and part of the total amount went back to the RNOH.

---

[124] For details of Charnley's development work, see Gomez and Morcuende (2005a and b). See also Foreman-Peck (1995); Dorr *et al.* (2000); Bechtol (1973).

[125] See note 87.

Lettin: It didn't go to the individual as it would now.

Dowson: Chairman, just one or two brief comments. You mentioned earlier, and reference has been made in the discussion, to a number of significant meetings of the BOA and other organizations. I would like to remind people that in the engineering field, a joint meeting between the Institution of Mechanical Engineers (IMechE) and the BOA was held in 1967. I think that this was a landmark in many ways, and John Charnley was on the planning committee of four people, as was John Scales; they were the two representatives from the BOA. When I look through the list of contributors, it reads like a *Who's Who* of joint replacement history, on both the engineering and on the surgical side.

Mike Freeman raised a point earlier as did, I think, Alan Swanson, which made me wonder about the way in which polyethylene replaced PTFE, since it appeared that there was some knowledge available at that time of the ill effects of radiation. It was a different era of information technology. Because in the same way as when John Charnley was introducing PTFE, engineers knew very well that it was a terrible material for wear. It had the lowest known coefficient of friction for man-made materials, but manufacturers steered away from it as a bearing material in bulk form. I could never understand quite what persuaded John to go down that route. PTFE nearly always had to be strengthened as a bearing material for high loads. It had to be impregnated into metal, or involved in some other way, to be an effective bearing material. I think this point was important at that stage, alongside the irradiation issue.[126] And finally, just to say something about the discussion of surface replacement joints which seem to be attracting so much attention at the present stage, in metal-on-metal form. From the engineering point of view, it is very interesting that they would all have difficulty with small diameters, because up to about 28mm or 30mm diameter, they are always rubbing one material on the other, all the time; they are rubbing bearings. When you go to a larger diameter, 36mm and certainly up to 50mm or so, then you start to get some very important contributions to load support from the lubrication, which you do not get at lower diameters. This is having a big effect on the resurgence of interest in (a) large diameter metal-on-metal, and (b) resurfacing approaches. Much of the current work is, as yet, theoretical and experimental, and has, of course, to be substantiated in practice. One of the difficulties is that we are going to have to wait so very long before we see the outcome of clinical performance of these very low-wear-rate joint replacements.

---

[126] See note 7 and discussion on pages 37, 38, 50 and 57.

Sweetnam: I wanted to give Sir Christopher [Booth] an answer to his question. He asked whether all this work was being carried out in an international vacuum. Let us go forth from this meeting knowing that it was. This was a British innovative idea – British surgeons, materials, scientists, engineers – conceived the practical concept of total hip replacement. What you are talking about – why it [control of the industry] eventually moved to the US later – occurs after the events that we are considering today.[127] This was a British initiative carried forward with great success. So that is the answer.

Booth: Thank you very much.

Freeman: I am very moved by Rodney's view, but I do not think we should absolutely ignore the contribution of others. I'm not quite sure what this meeting today is about: UK joint replacement, or hip replacement?

Lettin: Basically it is total hip replacement, UK. It is really Rodney's view of life, I think.

Freeman: It is perfectly all right that we mention Maurice Müller and some of these other people?[128] [Yes.] The second question is that, although we are wonderful to have invented this [total hip replacement], we made a terrible industrial disaster. As an industry, it is entirely dominated by the US. I wonder whether anyone would like to comment on that part of the subject?

Lettin: I don't know. It is certainly dominated by the US, there is only one British company now in the business and that is Smith and Nephew, isn't it.[129] Minuscule.

Booth: But they are only jokingly English. It's the business, really – the only ones in the business are Americans.

---

[127] Dr Francis Neary wrote: 'It was really manufacturing control that moved to the US when the small UK companies were mostly bought out by the US giants Zimmer, DePuy (later Johnson & Johnson), Biomet, Howmedica (later Stryker Howmedica) and Smith and Nephew (which retains a British connection)'. E-mail to Mrs Lois Reynolds, 15 October 2006.

[128] Maurice Müller of Bern introduced a femoral prosthesis that had a high rate of stem breakages and was fabricated from cast cobalt–chrome alloy with a curved shape. Müller's later stem had a 32mm head and was called the Charnley-Müller prosthesis. Klenerman (2002): 17. See also Schmalzried *et al.* (1996).

[129] Foreman-Peck (1995).

Lettin: But they can't get the FDA to approve the McMinn.[130] I don't want to get into that, but Smith and Nephew's head office is in the UK, but the real action is in the US.

Kirkup: In 1915 the disposable surgical blade was introduced in the US. When the patent ran out in 1930 or thereabouts, Swann-Morton of Sheffield took it over. And now, Swann-Morton is worldwide, the biggest manufacturer of blades, even supplying large areas of the US.[131]

Heywood-Waddington: In response to the comments on the British contribution, I have to say that with the recent progress since then in litigation and politics, I very much doubt whether Charnley and McKee would have succeeded in this day and age in their endeavours, it took so long. We owe a great deal, not only to their tenacity, but to the political and social side of the prevailing climate.

Kunzru: A question concerns the approach to children's hips, because many of them were quite deformed. George Arden always took off the trochanter to do his hip replacements, his custom-built hips, but you [Swann] didn't. Would you like to talk about your approach, please.

Swann: The approach I used to these hips, which were all anatomically deformed, varied, but was basically the lateral approach. That was my favourite. Occasionally it was necessary to remove the trochanter, just from the technical approach point of view, not from any other reason, just to get at the joint.

Lettin: We'll stop now for tea. I hope the films and videos will be ready to view at your leisure. Thank you, you've all been very good. Francis Neary will start the post-tea session from a historical point of view.

Dr Francis Neary: I wanted to say a bit about the roots of the proposal of this seminar, and the research we have been doing in Manchester, because some of the people here might be interested in some of its products. This project was led by Professor John Pickstone and was called 'Innovation, Assessment and Hip Prosthesis'. We looked at the work of Sir John Charnley, especially his relationship with Thackray, but also the development of the clean-air operating

---

[130] Mr Alan Lettin wrote: 'I believe that the McMinn has since been approved by the FDA.' Note on draft transcript, 25 November 2006.

[131] Swann-Morton, founded in Sheffield in 1932, manufactures surgical blades, scalpels and handles. See www.swann-morton.com/ (visited 5 June 2006).

system, and the relationship with Howorth Air Conditioning.[132] We also considered two wider issues, and these were particularly relevant to this seminar today: the early local development of THR in the five centres that we have been discussing.[133] One other issue, which we may move on to later on, perhaps, is the issue we have alluded to: why so many designs of hip replacements are now available, and why not one won out over the 50 years that total hip replacement has been available? Why are there so many different prostheses on the market? Very quickly, turning to the book on the history of hip replacement written with my colleagues Julie Anderson and John Pickstone, which will be available next year, I believe, and a series of journal articles.[134] But more topically, there's a new exhibition which I have done with Simon Chaplin at the Royal College of Surgeons, called 'Hip Histories', and what it does is it looks at the Charnley hip from the perspective of the nurse, the engineer, the surgeon, the patient and the manufacturer, and looks at its development. That's on the second floor of the Royal College of Surgeons' Hunterian Museum in the temporary gallery, called the Qvist Gallery.[135] And the other thing that I just wanted briefly to say is that we are also developing a patient information centre at Wrightington Hospital, which will open at the end of the month [March 2006] and has been generously supported by the John Charnley Trust. It will use history to explain the risks, benefits and unknowns of joint replacement surgery and take the patient from initial referral to the hospital, right the way through to surgery and recovery. And the plan is to also open a new Charnley Museum at Wrightington, sometime later in the summer.

Lettin: Thank you very much, Francis. One of the themes of research that Sir Christopher [Booth] mentioned to me over tea was that these innovations in orthopaedics, and probably in other fields too, have come not from academic centres, but from part-time NHS consultants, working in District General Hospitals. I suppose this is not quite true of the Royal National Orthopaedic Hospital (RNOH) at Stanmore, although many people would regard it as a

---

[132] For the background of the Howorth firm, see note 24.

[133] Development of the total hip replacment began in Norwich (between 1940–51); Stanmore (1956); Wrightington (1956); Redhill (1964) and Exeter (1969). See note 6.

[134] See Anderson *et al.* (forthcoming, 2007); Anderson (2006); Pickstone (2006); Metcalfe and Pickstone (2006). For details of the Manchester hip project, see www.york.ac.uk/res/iht/projects/l218252045.htm (visited 23 May 2006).

[135] For details of the exhibition, see www.hero.ac.uk/uk/culture___sport/archives/2006/radical_surgery.cfm (visited 3 January 2007).

general hospital. I know it did have pretensions at one time of being an academic centre, but I think this is interesting, isn't it? Sir Christopher felt that this was certainly something that should be part of the record.

But having said that, I think the next topic that we put down on paper, was the question of complications, because of course no operation, in spite of what one might hope, is ever going to be free of complications, and I suppose we did mention earlier the question of dislocation. That in some ways, I think, goes with the operative technique, and we might go on to that in a bit. The first thing that we should address is the question of mechanical failure, which was something that happened early on, but perhaps as a result of the BSI controls is not as common as it once was. What about the engineers, Alan, would you like to say anything about mechanical failure and the design? Was the design responsible, perhaps, or was it a question of manufacturing, or what?

Swanson: I could say a lot or little, I should prefer the latter, and no doubt you will too. I suspect that most of the mechanical failures, in the sense of the thing breaking, were due to the manufacture of the metal components. I think nowadays people just don't make cobalt chromium alloys with the kind of segregation of alloy elements to grain boundaries, which did happen 50 years ago. The composition of the so-called stainless steel has been refined enormously over the years, and again things are added or carbon contents get lower and so on and so forth. All sorts of things have been done to reduce the susceptibility to crevice corrosion for example, so I strongly suspect that we should now see far, far fewer breakages of the components, mainly because of attention to manufacture. It's still possible for the surgeon to put the thing in less than the optimum alignment, for example, which might have an effect on cup migration and all sorts of things. But I strongly suspect that attention to the metal alloys and the manufacturing thereof is what really has made the difference.

And while I am speaking, I would like to mention another point. The thing that would impress me most is long-term comparisons of different procedures. Of course, as soon as I start to say this, everybody else here knows at least as well as I do that one can't compare one procedure against another because too many variables are involved. And so as an engineer, I am repeatedly frustrated if anybody asks me, as they sometimes do, 'I am going to hospital to have my hip replaced, what do you recommend?' I have to say, 'I am sorry, the data, as far as I know, does not exist, where one could separate the effect of the prostheses' designs, prostheses' materials, the surgeon's technique, the patient selection, and so on and so forth.' And I fully realize that it would be an enormous task, but it seems to me that there is an enormous gap in the knowledge we have available that would shed light on what to do. Any engineer can look at any prosthesis and think of a reason why it might fail, but what really matters is how often it does fail and when.

Lettin: I think we are coming to that, certainly when we talk about results and follow-up. That is something which one should be able to answer and I think there has been a move forward, and I know it does seem that three or four prostheses seem to have been going for a sufficiently long time, with sufficient numbers to be able to make some assessment.[136]

Wroblewski: May I make a comment for the record. Between 1962 and 1968 – the beginning of the Charnley LFA – 2500 were carried out at Wrightington Hospital. There was not a single revision for a loose cup, a loose or fractured stem: six years, 2500 operations. The first fractured stem appeared in 1968. The main problem was a loss, or lack of, proximal stem support, and bending torsion. A loose stem followed, and finally wear and loosening of the cup.[137] So, no problems in six years and 2500 operations. The information we have available has passed 30 years now and it makes fascinating reading. But to say that information is not available, is incorrect. Secondly, my dear sir, if you are worried, pick yourself a good surgeon.

Older: Just to pick up, you were asking about complications in the early days. I have been reviewing Charnley's low-friction arthroplasties as performed by Charnley himself from 1970–74, that is nearly 300 LFAs, and some patients are still alive and I still see them. In that series, there has been 6 per cent with fractures of the stem of the femoral component. Michael Wroblewski has bigger figures and has looked at this in greater depth. Of the 6 per cent of fractures – some of them even fractured 20 years after Charnley put them in – but I am told that since 1982, when the manufacturers started using Ortron,[138] there hasn't been a single fracture of the femoral stem. That is an indication of a technical complication associated, not entirely as Michael perhaps suggests, on the loading, but I think it was also a reflection of the nature of the metal that was being used by Charnley.

---

[136] See Table 1 on page 75.

[137] Charnley (1975a and b); Decoulx (1975); Olsson *et al.* (1981); Wroblewski (1986, 1990); Pacheco *et al.* (1988).

[138] Ortron 90 is the brand name used by DePuy International Ltd, Leeds, for ISO/5832-9 stainless steel. See Appendix 2 for early ISO standards.

Lettin: So the materials are obviously very important.

Stephen: As many of you will know, but for the record: in the early Exeter experience, there were a series of both stem and neck breakages due to manufacturing errors. Firstly, the material used in the stem, and later, overmachining of the neck, led to fatigue failure. I would support the contention of the engineers; this is a feature of the manufacturing process.

Lettin: Will the BSI overcome this, will standards cover so that this shouldn't happen in the future?

Wheble: There had been work done on this subject for the BSI committee. It was endurance testing to see what was happening to prostheses under load. The rigs used examined two problems: the effects of torsion applied to the prosthesis when under varying load and extended time; and the effects of various loads when applied directly to the ball of the prosthesis with the neck unsupported but the stem firmly fixed. These tests were continued for long periods of time, but as far as I am aware, they never resulted in the writing of a standard for tests of this type.

Lettin: But the manufacturers test them all now. They are tested in batches presumably, Phyllis, not individually.

Hampson: Our manufactured items were sent weekly to Stanmore for checking before we were allowed to have them back, repack, and sterilize and then sell them.

Lettin: Does anybody know whether every individual implant is tested against these standards, or just batches?

Hampson: There's no 'you must check' recurrence. That doesn't come into it. We agreed because that's what John Scales wanted and we thought it was a good thing, but I think now this doesn't happen. I really don't believe that every company tests batches of prostheses.

Swanson: On this question of testing, Chairman, one can measure each individual prosthetic component, for example one can do the surface finish, but when it comes to fatigue testing, or corrosion testing, it can only be done on a sample basis, and there are well known techniques in industries where these things matter, like aeroplanes, which I used to be in, where there are immense procedures, all laid down, about the frequency of sampling, and what you do if one isn't quite right, and so on. I think we should understand that with joint prostheses, as with cars and aeroplanes, and everything else, we are putting our faith in statisticians.

Hampson: That's probably true to a great extent. But we also had an agreement with Stanmore that we would keep samples of all the materials used up to seven years, so that if Stanmore found a hip prosthesis on their test machine that wasn't working properly, or it broke or whatever, we had to go through the whole of the numbering system and clear every prosthesis out of stock and check through the materials of the samples we kept.

Lettin: But I am right in concluding that although we have these standards, there is no obligation on the manufacturers to meet these standards? This is a very unsatisfactory state of affairs, isn't it, Rodney?

Sweetnam: Yes, but it may have changed now.[139]

Lettin: At least I know that you agree with me anyway. Yes, so mechanical failure: is there anything that you would like to say, Duncan, about mechanical failure?

Dowson: The only additional thing I would say is that a lot of the implant performance characteristics which you may wish to know do not readily emerge from standard simulator tests. If you are going to evaluate whether or not a given total hip replacement is satisfactory from the point of view of wear, it may be necessary to spend six months on a simulator, for each implant design, and this is both restrictive and expensive. You have to rely on statistical methods for both laboratory and clinical evaluations, sooner or later. Few current simulators replicate the daily cycles of loads and motions to which implants are exposed *in vivo*.

Freeman: A point of order, Chairman, under mechanical failure, do you include wear? Or are you just talking about fracture? You are only talking about one of the two components.

Lettin: I was going to talk about wear next, if that's all right. I was actually going to say that a definition of a statistician is a chap who when you ask him how his wife is, he says, 'Compared with whom?' [Laughter] Perhaps we should move on to wear. Would you start the ball rolling, Michael?

---

[139] See note 65.

Freeman: I would like to know from the regulators who we have here, what the requirements are for the polyethylene component: are they scrutinized in any way, on a batch basis, before they go out? Would it be possible, for example, to know how much oxygen they had in them, how cross-linked they were, etc.? And it has been said, I believe, that wear was the major problem. I wonder whether we agree, as historians looking back, that the major problem was due to the fact not that the high-density polyethylene polymer components were polyethylene, but because with some exceptions they were gamma-irradiated in air, they came to the market to a certain extent as, actually, a low-molecular weight polyethylene. Are we scrutinizing the polyethylene? Have we made a mistake in the past?

Lettin: I don't know. Phyllis, were you scrutinizing the polyethylene?

Hampson: No, we weren't. We used to visit the manufacturers in Germany every six months to ensure that we knew what they were doing, but of course they repeatedly changed the formula without telling anybody, so you couldn't really check the polyethylene at all.

From the floor: So you had no idea what this stuff was?

Hampson: No.

Ms Clare Darrah: I am sorry there is nobody here from industry today, but I think in their defence they do comply with very stringent European standards and now, certainly, with the ISO/9000.[140] Quite what they all mean is a bit of a mystery to me, but I think we should be a little careful to say that they are not complying.

Tucker: May I confirm that. If you ask the so-called experts, they will say that there are European standards for pretty well everything, including surface finish, high-density polyethylene, etc. [see Appendix 2]. Companies will declare their standards, and if you challenge them they will say that they have quality control, and that they are manufacturing to the standard. From what I have gleaned, standards are quite lax. Take surface finish, for example, particularly on HDP acetabulae, the range offered by European Directives is quite wide.

---

[140] ISO/9000 (2000) is a generic name given to a group of standards developed by the British Standards Institution that provide a quality management system framework to ensure consistency and improvement of working practices. It claims to be the most commonly used international standard for an effective quality management. See www.bsi-emea.com/Quality/Overview/WhatisISO9000.xalter (visited 14 November 2006).

Lettin: There's certainly no obligation for the standards to be met, but if it's not met, and there was some problem, then of course litigation, compensation, would be multiplied considerably, I would imagine.

Tucker: They have to obey the European standard.

Lettin: But we don't know how carefully they test their products. But that would be in their contract.

Swanson: A very brief point, I don't think one should shelter too confidently behind the ISO/9000 series. My friends, who are still active in engineering industry, tell me this is more about the firm's general procedures and the integrity of its filing system, than about actually looking at the product. I could tell you a horror story about a bus that was falling to pieces, run by a company that is accredited to ISO/9000, but I won't.

Wroblewski: I think I would like to ask Professor Swanson a question. You have done some work with Barry Weightman on the quality of the high-molecular weight polyethylene, examining explanted Charnley cups with a follow-up of 17 years.[141] Perhaps you would be kind enough to remind us what the results were?

Swanson: I know I am getting old and my memory is failing. I have no memory whatever of myself or Barry Weightman handling an explanted Charnley cup. I think you may mean Professor Dowson.

Wroblewski: No, the two of you [Weightman and Swanson] looked at wear and degradation, examining the worn and the unworn parts of the cup, matching specimens, and testing them for wear characteristics. The conclusion was that there was no evidence of batch-to-batch variation or degradation of the material in the human body.

Swanson: I suppose I had better go home and look up my own publication list. I am sorry I have no memory at all of this.

Lettin: Anybody else? We are still on the subject of wear.

Dr Alex Faulkner: Sorry, not quite on the subject of wear, but we shouldn't leave the topic of standards without mentioning that hip implants have just (in 2005) been reclassified under European Directives as a grade 3 rather than

---

[141] Weightman *et al.* (1991).

a grade 2B device, which means that clinical evidence will be required for new prostheses in all cases, which hasn't been the case before.[142]

Lettin: Yes, there are obviously very great difficulties from an orthopaedic point of view we only really know when they go wrong, and that is after a period of time often, and these directives they end after a year or something don't they, Keith? You only have to provide one year of follow-up or something.

Tucker: That is the case with the CE mark, but fortunately in this country we have now managed to loop the political problems of 'post-market surveillance' and we have National Institute for Health and Clinical Excellence (NICE) guidelines. NICE commissioned the NHS Purchasing and Supply Agency to set up the Orthopaedic Data Evaluation Panel (ODEP), which is run by Andy Smallwood with myself as Chairman.[143] This means for a product to be sold in the UK the implant has to have a rating. Thus, post-market surveillance is still not around, as such, but if a manufacturer wishes to sell an implant to a private hospital in the UK or into the NHS, the implant must have a benchmark. The ideal benchmark is 10A, which the Charnley, the Exeter and the Stanmore, together with quite a few overseas and newer prostheses,[144] have acquired. If you develop a new product you go into pre-entry (which is not a benchmark) and then move through the three-, five- and seven-year benchmarks before acquiring a 10A. During the progression to 10A the company will have to collect data on its implant and satisfy the ODEP criteria. Thus we have looped the European nuisance of not allowing post-market surveillance by having this facility. The ODEP panel works closely with the National Joint Registry and the idea is to catch out prostheses which don't work.[145] Michael [Wroblewski], I know you are

---

[142] Dr Alex Faulkner wrote: 'European Commission Directive 2005/50/EC of 11 August 2005 on the reclassification of hip, knee and shoulder joint replacements in the framework of Council Directive 93/42/EEC concerning medical devices. *Official Journal of the European Union*, 12 August 2005, L210/41–3.' E-mail to Mrs Lois Reynolds, 10 October 2006.

[143] For further details, see www.pasa.nhs.uk/medical/orthopaedics/odepdatabase/ (visited 1 August 2006); see also NICE (2000).

[144] See Appendix 3, pages 101–06.

[145] The National Joint Registry was launched in April 2003. The contract to establish it was awarded to AEA Technology in September 2002, managed by a Steering Committee chaired by Bill Darling CBE and vice chaired by Professor Paul Gregg, then President of the BOA [DoH Press Release 2003/0146]. Northgate Information Solutions took over the management of the contract from April 2006. For further details, see the DoH website at www.dh.gov.uk/Home/fs/en (visited 14 November 2006).

thinking that we have a long way to go, and I am sure you are quite right, but I think we are getting a bit further forward.[146]

Lettin: This is bringing us up to date, but historically we are going on in a minute to follow-up and I mean this is really all we have at the moment, is long-term follow-up, isn't it? We haven't really got away from wear.

Dowson: Just a comment on that, Chairman. The typical wear rate in volumetric terms is, of course, generally related to the polyethylene, the UHMWPE, which is perhaps 30 to 50 cubic millimetres a year. If you now move to a well-designed metal-on-metal implant – and one reason for this being done is to minimize the wear volume, because of the osteolysis [bone loss] problem with polyethylene wear debris – then the wear in the first year or two might be 1 or 2 cubic millimetres, and thereafter less than one tenth of a cubic millimetre per year. The question is related not to just the volume of wear, but the nature of the wear debris. And although the wear rate of the metal-on-metal is so much lower – impressively lower than that of the polyethylene from the metal-on-polymer configuration – the size of the metallic particles of the metal-on-metal joint wear debris is so very small, that there are several times as many metallic wear particles as there are polyethylene particles generated each year. And the question is what do these particles do in terms of biological reaction and the jury seems to be out on this, as I think Mike Freeman was saying earlier.[147] There may be cause for concern, superficially, but we are awaiting the hard evidence.

Lettin: This really does bring us on to the real problem of wear. From an ordinary layman's point of view, the recipient of the hip replacement is concerned whether

---

[146] Mr Keith Tucker wrote: 'My recollection is that in spite of provisional recommendations by Charnley, and later on by Mr Robin Ling in the mid-1980s, the DoH would not heed our suggestion of a hip registry. When I joined the MDA (MHRA) there seemed to be complete opposition to the idea of a registry. It was the National Audit Office [(2000)] that recommended a hip registry in their report on the Capital hip replacement debacle. This was in the mid-1990s when NICE also supported the concept of a hip registry. To many of us it was sad that the DoH's attitude towards a hip registry was so negative for so long. It stated in the Capital hip registry report that a hip registry had been in place at the time of the introduction of the Capital hip [see note 198] the problems may well not have occurred, or at least have been less widespread.' Fax to Mrs Lois Reynolds, 28 November 2006. See National Audit Office (2003), which notes that by this time 11 per cent of hip replacements used prostheses without adequate evidence of effectiveness, and 1 in 10 orthopaedic consultants prioritized patients on the basis of the need to meet waiting list targets.

[147] See the special issue on the development of monolithic and surface replacement metal-on-metal hip replacements in the *Proceedings of the Institution of Mechanical Engineers. Part H, Journal of Engineering in Medicine* 220[H2]: 1–407. See also Willert *et al.* (1974); Willert and Semlitsch (1976).

it will wear out. But that isn't really the problem. The problem is, as you have highlighted, the effects of the products of wear and this is not really new, this is old, isn't it? You were pointing out in that first historical period, that we are supposed to be considering – I don't know whether we have exceeded our brief in talking about current issues – Michael Freeman was talking about the effect on the DNA. Your original paper, Michael, as far as I remember, was on the carcinogenic effects of the wear products.[148] It was his paper, not yours. [**From the floor:** You shared it? **Freeman:** Yes, F [Freeman] comes before S [Swanson] in those titles.] But this was known in the period that we are talking about, the 1950s, 1960s, 1970s.

Freeman: May we read the name Hans Willert into the record. I know he is not English, he was German and worked in Switzerland, but he put the particle pathology business on the map in the early 1970s.[149] So it's not new, and we could have reduced the wear rate – I don't want to harp on this – by understanding the effects of irradiation on the polyethylene. It is not only that the manufacturers kept making different stuff [polyethylene] and supplying it to the implant makers, but the implant makers then sterilized it, and sent it off in batches, to be gamma-irradiated in air.

Lettin: And then left it on the shelves for several months.

Freeman: And then left it on the shelf, but everybody was doing it. We were collectively ignorant of the physical consequences of doing that to polyethylene, and Mike Wroblewski and Duncan know much more about this than I do, but it was a major problem that has been hidden under the carpet, because the medico–legal consequences of taking it out from under the carpet don't bear thinking about.

Wroblewski: Although what you say, Mike [Freeman], is partly correct, there is another issue. The main problem of cup-loosening is penetration, restricting angular movement by impingement. If you put off the moment of impingement by reducing the diameter of the neck, as it is possible to do with the Charnley stem in Ortron from 12.5mm to 10mm, you increase the range of movement by 18°. You do not generate any fewer wear particles. But over the 22 years that it has taken me to do this study, there is a reduction in the failure of cup

---

[148] Swanson *et al.* (1973).

[149] See, for example, Willert (1977); Semlitsch *et al.* (1977); Semlitsch and Willert (1997).

fixation of 56 per cent. So, although the volume of plastic shed into the tissues has increased, the incidence of cup loosening, radiologically and on revision, has been reduced by 56 per cent. I have spent some time with Professor Hans Willert of Gottingen, looking through his histology slides. I have histology slides with PTFE showing calcification and new bone formation.[150] Professor Willert accepts the evidence as a healing process. We do not know the full story. We cannot put it all down to just wear particles and tissue reaction to wear particles. That is not the full story.

Lettin: I think this really brings us on to the question of loosening, doesn't it, and really this is what you are saying. There's not just one cause of loosening, and perhaps we should explore that now. You are suggesting in fact that it's operative fault that can lead to loosening?

Wroblewski: There are two problems: one is failure of geometry, and we call it arthritis and for that we do hip replacement, and the second problem we 'create' is fixation of components. I wonder how many common-or-garden orthopaedic surgeons actually know to what loads the hip joint is subjected.[151] The BSI would not accept five times body weight as a standard for testing femoral components.

Heywood-Waddington: Could I be enlightened on that?

Lettin: Who's going to enlighten you?

Freeman: The answer is no, I don't have any evidence and I don't think there is any evidence, Mike. As far as I know there are a series of well-founded theoretical anxieties, but it's a bit like smoking, it takes a lot of years, and I would be very surprised if the theoretical anxieties manifested themselves in a population of people over the age of 60. They might do, but I would be very surprised, and certainly the fertility anxieties on the whole, I shouldn't think would, at that age, at least I hope to God they wouldn't, but it's when you get the younger people being hit by a lifetime of raised cobalt and chromium, then it might be different. Might, might not, I don't know, but it's an issue. While I am on this issue, I entirely agree with Mike Wroblewski, obviously, that the impingement issue of the lip of the acetabulum is a big thing, and you asked me why resurfacing arthroplasty failed and that is one reason – the head–neck ratio

---

[150] Wroblewski *et al.* (1995).

[151] See note 170.

is all wrong – and if you put in a 180° cup, you can hardly move it at all, before something bangs on something else.

Lettin: Design fault.

Wroblewski: Maybe we should ask a different question to answer the problem of tissue reaction to various metals. Maybe we should ask what are the recommended blood levels for these metals?

Lettin: I don't know if anybody knows.

Sweetnam: The answer is, as Michael Freeman has said, that nobody knows and will not know for very many years, because this is a long-term potential worry. But I think the message that should go from this group, of people who have experience of the development of hip replacement over the last 30 years or so, is that we, in 2006, are still very concerned about the absence of clear surveillance of new prostheses and new techniques, particularly large head metal-on-metal, and the fears – the theoretical fears – that we all know may or may not, as Michael [Freeman] has said, lead to serious complications at the end of the road. I think that is the message that we should be giving. I like to think that somebody may be listening. We should say that we, as a group, are worried about the future, the lack of surveillance and the long-term effects of released metal ions, particularly in those having metal-on-metal implants at an early age. That's my proposition, but maybe people don't agree.

Lettin: It will be recorded, Rodney. What do we think the main reason is in everyday practice for loosening? Do we think it is malposition of the components, in other words bad operative techniques? Is it bad cementing techniques, or is it these terrible wear particles? What's the feeling about this? What is the most significant cause of loosening? Does anybody know?

Wroblewski: I am very fortunate because I have access to information going back to November 1962. If the failure occurs in the first six years, i.e. loosening of the cup or loosening of the stem, in absence of infection, the problem is almost always technical. From then onwards, it is wear of the cup and loosening of the cup. After 12 to 14 years on the femoral side, it is proximal strain shielding.

Lettin: I think everybody knows that you have got very careful follow-up at Wrightington. Does anybody else have a comment? What about Ian Stephen for Robin Ling? He very carefully follows up all his patients, as I understand it.

Stephen: Yes, indeed, the follow-up has been meticulous and he feels that he has overcome the problem of stem loosening by the combination of stem geometry and cementing technology due to the behaviour of the double taper straight polished stem, which is self-tightening, and self-adjusting under load.

Lettin: Have you any comment on that, Michael?

Wroblewski: I quite agree with Ian, I think we have got to look on the femoral side. The design and the surgical technique must employ the common engineering principles that of male and female tapers engaging under load. For that system to become load-bearing, there must be a slip. That slip must be of the stem within the cement mantle. The question now concerns the stem design, surface finish, and the surgical technique. The problem from then onwards is bending torsion. We project ourselves, while walking, upwards and forwards, not just forwards, so the rotation is downwards and backwards. It is the proximal stem support which is important, so I entirely agree with Ian.

Lettin: Any other comments on the question of loosening, of how we can minimize it? I suppose we will never prevent it.

Freeman: May I support Rodney Sweetnam on the issue of surveillance, because here we are, a bunch of old men looking back at the 1960s and 1970s; we have 30 or 40 years of experience of this, and actually, Chairman, we can't answer your question, which is why do these damn things fail? The Swedes can. Apparently we are supposed to confine ourselves to the UK, but the Swedes have got a reasonable data system in Sweden,[152] which enables them to answer your question, but we don't know the answer.

Lettin: What is their answer?

Freeman: There's a thing called the Swedish hip survey which I suppose depends on the personality of Sweden and its size and the population and one thing and another.[153] But unless we have such a thing here, and I actually can't imagine how we would ever get it into operation. If we have this meeting in 20 years time, we still couldn't answer your question.

---

[152] Ahnfelt *et al.* (1990); Malchau (1996). All failures after total hip arthroplasty in Sweden have been recorded since 1979 using medical records from every implant and revision, which were documented and computer analyzed.

[153] Malchau (1996).

Implant: cup & stem	Period	No. of implants	7-year survival %	10-year survivial %
Exeter mixed [154]	1980–1995	3758	97.0	94.9
Charnley	1979–2000	38 769	94.7	92.0
Stanmore	1979–1998	1549	96.2	91.9
Exeter matt	1980–1986	2623	92.1	86.2

Table 1: Survival rates of Charnley, Stanmore and Exeter THR.
Extracted from the Swedish Total Hip Replacement Register of 118 572 hips implanted between 1979–2000, arranged by 10-year survival rate.
Malchau *et al.* (2002): 9, Table 1

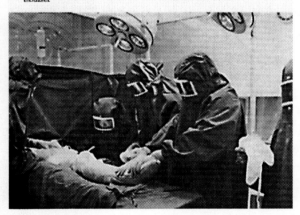

Comparative Figures compiled by the Pathological Department Wrightington Hospital

System	Year	Colonies/plate/hr.	Total No. of Operations	Infection %
Conventional theatre with exhaust ventilation	1959–1961	80-90	190	8.9
First prototype enclosure Electro-static filter	1962	26	108	3.7
Second prototype Howorth donated system	1963–1965	1.8	1079	2.2
Howorth Permanent Enclosure Mk. 1	1966–1968	0 (limit of accuracy)	1929	1.5
Howorth Permanent Enclosures Mk. I & Mk. II and	1969–1970* 1971–1972	0	2152 over 2000	0.5 0.3
Howorth Demountable System Type DF10	1973–1976	0	over 4000	0.3

Total to end 1976 11,783 operations

* Total Body Exhaust System was introduced only in the second half of 1970, in all enclosures.

Figure 24: Howorth publicity literature on the influence of the clean-air enclosure (the inside of the enclosure is shown here) and the surgeons' full-body exhaust suit, c. 1976.

[154] The Exeter stems were polished from 1970–75; matt: 1975–86; polished monolithic: 1986–88 and modular polished (Exeter Universal) from 1988 on. The data shown here between 1980–95 has both matt and polished stems.

Older: This is a comment, because I don't have an answer. But we are now looking at what I feel is the very guts of the longevity of a prosthesis, the interface between the prosthesis – whatever it is – and the patient's tissue. The interface is a combination of a mechanical and a biological relationship: mechanical in terms of the prosthesis that has been put in, and the method of the entry of that prosthesis chosen by the surgeon. And then there is the biological relationship: how the body reacts at that interface, because of what has been put in mechanically. Isn't it true that in those very few moments that the surgeon puts the prosthesis in, both he and the patient are going to govern the longevity of the prosthesis. So there is a very important mechanical aspect. One of John Charnley's favourite sayings was: 'Mechanical process is far more important than metallurgy'. Of course, the composition of the prosthesis is important, but it is this combination of mechanical and biological behaviour at the interface that is going to determine whether that prosthesis lasts one year or 20 or 30 years. The factors that affect that are very multi-factorial and, as Michael Freeman and Michael Wroblewski have said, we still haven't got the answer.

Lettin: All these things were known in this period that we are supposed to be discussing: the second half of the twentieth century and even earlier. We still don't know the answer. We are supposed to be discussing the early development, and I suppose we have drifted a bit from that, but these problems were known, and they haven't been resolved. What about infection? That was certainly known, and who was it, somebody said John Charnley's original infection rate was something like 6 per cent? [**From the floor:** Nearly 9 per cent.] [See Figure 24]

We have heard a bit about the greenhouse, and this was a very big thing at one stage, wasn't it? The DoH was very much concerned whether the cost of introducing, building, or putting clean air theatres into hospitals, and all the rest of it, was cost-effective. This was a very big thing, and I think there was a study by the MRC,[155] of where the infection came from, and to my recollection a chap came to the BOA and told us that it all emanated from the perineum of the surgeons and the nurses and the immediate consequences of that was that nurses no longer wore dresses in theatres, but wore trousers. It didn't seem to me that that stopped the appropriately offending bacteria from descending the trouser leg. And I thought I would carry this to its conclusion and I went to the theatre one day and tied string around my trousers just below the knee, which looked rather like those pictures you see of labourers in the fields in

---

[155] DHSS and MRC, Joint Working Party (1972).

the nineteenth century and it caused considerable hilarity among the theatre staff, but the next day my anaesthetist went one better and came in wearing cycle clips on his trousers. I suppose the clean air theatre and the exhaust tubes were really eliminating expired air, which the MRC study, as I understand it, demonstrated was not a great source of bacteria.[156]

Wroblewski: Up-currents, skin scales, those are also important, not just exhaled air.

Lettin: No, but the MRC study, as I understand it, showed [that the source of the bacteria] was overwhelmingly from the perineum. Does nobody remember? [Much laughter.] Who was the chap at the BOA, who gave the talk, was it Lowrie or Lourie?[157]

Freeman: I have nothing to contribute except that skin scales, and the perineum are relevant, but not the end of the story.

Sweetnam: May I just raise one point. I keep on harking back to this business of somebody reading this discussion in 50 or 100 years' time, and I think one of the things that we ought to discuss is the question of the relevance of clean air. Now we all accepted as gospel that clean air is responsible for the reduction of sepsis. Is that so? At the same time that clean air was introduced, prophylactic antibiotics were also introduced and became widespread, and that was the recognized fallacy of the study of that time into the efficacy of clean air. So has the drop in infection in total hip replacements been due to clean air, which is widely used at vast expense, or prophylactic antibiotics?[158] I don't know the answer, maybe somebody else does.

Lettin: Didn't the MRC do a multi-centre trial, which included Sweden, and they couldn't get enough patients to make any significant conclusions?

---

[156] Lidwell *et al.* (1982). This is the first report on the MRC study of ultraclean air in 19 hospitals in England, Scotland and Sweden, 1975–79. The 4-year follow-up study of 8052 operations on hips and knees appears in Lidwell *et al.* (1987).

[157] Ted Lowbury. See Lidwell *et al.* (1982); Lowbury and Lidwell (1978); Lidwell *et al.* (1987).

[158] See note 169. Discussion of clean air versus antibiotics continued throughout the period. For example, a letter to the *BMJ* by the authors of the MRC study [Lidwell *et al.* (1983)] pointed out possible misleading conclusions drawn by Dr P D Meers' editorial, was printed along with Meers' reply [Meers (1983a and b)]. Freely available at Pub Med, see gateway at www.ncbi.nlm.nih.gov/entrez/query.fcgi?DB=pubmed (visited 22 November 2006).

Sweetnam: That is my point, it was done, but not [directly] by the MRC.[159] Actually it was inconclusive by scientific standards, because of the introduction of antibiotics at the same time. Indeed the authors admitted in their abstract that 'the design of the study did not include a strictly controlled test of the effect of prophylactic antibiotics'.[160]

Lettin: But they evaluated the antibiotics in that study, purely and simply. My recollection is that it was an improvement of ten times.[161]

Sweetnam: I am only talking about clean air, its value is likely but not entirely proven. There was criticism of the trial in the correspondence columns of the *British Medical Journal* (*BMJ*) later.[162]

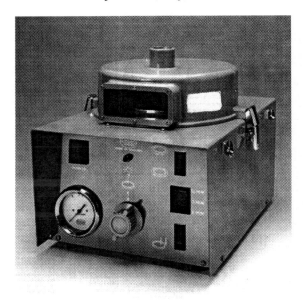

Figure 25: Casella slit sampler AIR14 used in the 1960 clean air enclosure, originally developed by the Medical Research Council. See Bourdillon *et al.* (1948): 15.

---

[159] Lowbury and Lidwell (1978); Lidwell *et al.* (1982). See note 156.

[160] Lidwell *et al.* (1982): 10.

[161] The number of patients being operated on in all conditions who did not receive antibiotics and whose implant had no sepsis was 2.3 per cent, compared to 0.6 per cent of those receiving antibiotics (flucloxacillin). Lidwell *et al.* (1982): 13, Table IV. See also Hill *et al.* (1981); Taggart *et al.* (2002).

[162] Meers (1983a). See note 158.

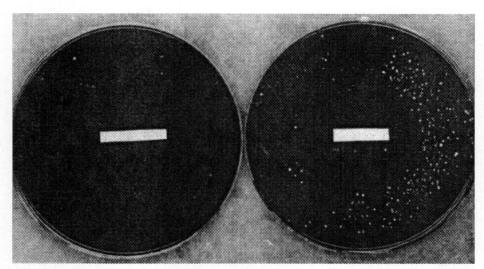

Figure 26: Two Petri dishes from a slit sampler with a rotation time of 60 minutes, c. 1960. Bacteria grown from air sampled: L. inside enclosure; R. outside enclosure.

Lady Charnley: If my memory serves me right, I remember very much that when that study came out John was absolutely delighted that it was agreeing with his figures, that clean air made a potential difference to infection. And I would also like to remind people that he developed the body exhaust system, which he found tremendously beneficial. I am afraid, I think it has gone out of fashion,[163] but it did have an enormous effect on the results of infection at Wrightington.

Lettin: It was very comfortable, in the sense that you had nice air.

Lady Charnley: He always said it was like operating on top of a mountain.

Mr Reg Elson: The MRC trial showed conclusively, as far as I am concerned, that there was a summation between the effects of systemic antibiotics and clean air.[164] At Wrightington the infection rate fell steeply with the introduction of the clean air enclosure, and without systemic antibiotics. There is no doubt that if, for example, you stand over a Petri dish in a clean-air enclosure and you wave your arms about in a sterile down-draught, you will get [bacterial] cultures.

---

[163] For a discussion of the recent decline of discipline in operating theatres, see S2C2 (2004a and b).

[164] Bourdillon *et al.* (1941, 1948); Blowers and Crew (1960); Lidwell and Williams (1960); Hughes (1988). The incidence of infection in hip replacement surgery from the MRC trial was less than 1 per cent in Lidwell *et al.* (1982). See note 156. See also Lidwell (1990).

Lettin: But all orthopaedic theatres are now clean-air theatres.

Elson: In the majority of cases replacements are done in clean air. But you see, illogically, some surgeons operate without a hood, only a cap, and the down-draught is actually dangerous.

Craven: When we were doing this work at Wrightington, I made a slit sampler that would run for one hour and we used to take readings all the time John Charnley was operating. We took readings on a 6-inch culture plate, so these could be sent to the lab, and check what bacteria were on it [see Figure 26]. I remember Charnley put John Read in a bag and had him wave his arms about, as this gentleman in front of me was doing, and if you had recently had a shower, the bacteria that came out was worse than if you hadn't, because all your pores were open.

Deane: The first clean-air enclosure outside Wrightington was set up at the Nuffield Orthopaedic Centre in Oxford, and I was responsible for commissioning this enclosure. It was all very splendid. There were quite a lot of running-in problems, getting it the way it was meant to be, because this was the first one outside Wrightington. The week after it was commissioned I wrote to Howorth, because of interest from a foreign visitor, who had seen these enclosures in use in this first week and liked the look of them. He expressed interest in possible supply to his country and I agreed to enquire for him. I had a letter back, the second sentence of which I will never forget. It said, approximately, 'We no longer supply the Howorth-type enclosure as your specification, as we consider it too costly for publicly-owned hospitals'. I still have that letter. Since that time, the excellent concept of clean-air theatres, including the body-exhaust system, has developed further. I am concerned that the development of clean-air enclosures has produced some with horizontal laminar flow, and some with vertical laminar flow, but the body-exhaust system has disappeared. I think this is actually producing worse conditions with the unsterile surgeon and other people standing in a beautiful blast of clean air and interrupting its flow over the patient, as Reg Elson has just said.[165]

Freeman: If you have vertical downflow and then you have to worry about the lighting of the operating table; unless they are very carefully cleaned, the lights

---

[165] While at the Nuffield Orthopaedic Centre, Mr Graham Deane undertook research on horizontal laminar air flow, photographing the air flow over the operating table and surgical team. The results were not published. For a discussion of the recent decline of discipline in operating theatres, see the Scottish Society for Contamination Control (S2C2) (2004).

are a source of dirt that is blown straight down into the wound, so the air is sterile at the roof, but it isn't on the level of the wound. Could you ask them, Mr Chairman, what is it that we are talking about? What is the infection rate now in the UK? As retired surgeons, we have no idea, I don't think, have we?

Wroblewski: 1.2 per cent over 32 years.

Freeman: No, not yours.

Wroblewski: Oh, I see.

Darrah: The Health Protection Agency now run mandatory data collection on one of three indicators in any hospital at any time: in neck of femur fractures, total hips, or total knee replacements. Data is collected for three months – and this is mandatory government surveillance, unlike the National Joint Registry.[166] This is how infection rates are known. The rates are published, and every hospital in the country has to supply the data in one of those three indications. So, depending on what indications you collect the data for, you have the infection rate for that indicator for that hospital.

Lettin: What about Norwich?

Darrah: The infection rate for total hip replacement at the moment is under 1 per cent.[167] The Health Protection Agency has a mandatory data collection for a three-month period, in any 12 months, and they collect the data during the operative stay, and up to six weeks post-operatively.

Lettin: It did drop to 1 per cent at one time, didn't it, in John Charnley's unit?

Wroblewski: Three months is not long enough. If you are talking about patients with deep infection after total hip arthroplasty, you need about four years to cover about 43 per cent revisions for deep infection. Deep infection, given time, will present itself, but it takes longer than nine months.

Lettin: So we are talking about really acute infections, the incidence of acute infection within the three months of the operation is 2 per cent.

Freeman: If you are saying that the infection rate in a very good hospital is under 2 per cent, which means it's above 1 per cent, nearly 2 per cent, within three months, and you multiply that by four or five to get the long-term figure,

---

[166] See note 145.

[167] Ms Clare Darrah wrote: 'For January–December 2005, 0.6 per cent'. Note on draft transcript, 3 July 2006.

we are looking at something like 8 per cent, 10 per cent infection rate, in the long term.

Elson: Also, there is another factor in this: the temporal sampling of three months, is totally inaccurate because these things go in bursts. What Mike was trying to say was that three months' sampling is a worthless measure of deep infection. Ninety per cent of deep infections will occur during the first year, but could come in any of the first three months, and they tend to come in bursts. You get bursts of infection, localized to about a week.

Professor John Pickstone: I was struck by the account of Charnley of working in an old hospital, in a theatre that was used by lots of other people. Is it the case that the infection was more of a problem at Wrightington than it was at other early centres, before clean-air enclosures spread?

Lettin: It was certainly regarded at the time as being quite high, wasn't it? And that was why John Charnley introduced the greenhouse.

Pickstone: Yes, I know that's why he introduced the greenhouse, but were his problems particularly severe because of where he was working, or was he simply the first person to get to grips with these problems?

Wroblewski: Because of different surgeons [using the same theatre].

Freeman: He was the first to get to grips with them.

Pickstone: I mean the problems of bad theatres were by no means confined to Wrightington. Were the infection rates at other early sites much the same as they were at Wrightington?

Freeman: They were much worse. There were birds flying around.

Tucker: I would like to touch on the historical aspect. I think that the concepts of 'deep infection' and 'superficial infection' (the words we use today) weren't terribly well defined in the late 1960s. Ken McKee would sometimes see a wound that was discharging, and he would say that it was a 'rejection'. I don't think we understood then what was going on. Swabs were taken and came back from the laboratory with reports of *Staphylococcus epidermidis,* coagulase negative *Staphylococcus,*[168] or perhaps a bowel organism. The laboratories were saying that these were either normal skin flora or contamination.

---

[168] *Staphylococcus epidermidis,* the most important of the coagulase negative staphylococci (CoNS), can cause infection in in-dwelling medical devices.

We now know that these organisms are an awful nuisance, and in hindsight they usually indicated the presence of a deep infection with a discharging sinus. At the time we were living with a view, emanating from many highly regarded bacteriology departments, that we shouldn't treat infection until we had isolated the organism. Some bacteriologists said that prophylactic antibiotics were totally out of order. I think it should go on record that orthopaedics taught bacteriology departments quite a bit around the late 1960s and early 1970s. One thing we haven't recorded in our discussion is the introduction of *Gentamicin*-impregnated cement following the work of Buchholz.[169] For many patients this made a lot of difference.

Lettin: That is really going back to our original terms of reference, so to speak, and we have moved on quite a bit. I think probably this would be the appropriate time to move on to revision before we finally wind up with results and follow-up. Reg [Elson], perhaps you would like to talk about revision, the most difficult cause of which was infection, but no doubt you will embrace all the reasons for revising things and how difficult it could be in mere mortals' hands.

Elson: I wondered what to say on the train coming down, and I am still wondering now. I have probably done as many revision hips and probably knees, as anybody else in the room. I have industrial deafness as a result of working with Charnley, that terrible noise of air rush against your eardrums: I am thinking of suing.

Now it's axiomatic that every hip will wear out, break, fall out, if the patient lives long enough. I am amazed that so many colleagues still will allow patients to do whatever they like in terms of physical activity; you see these glamorous photographs, in films, of people playing tennis or skiing. Recently I have done a study on the actual loading of the hip in certain postures, and if – as the Swiss do, they allow their patients to go skiing – the load that you can calculate on the hip, is way above anything [John] Paul taught us: about 5.8 x bodyweight for normal brisk walking, ten times body weight, quite apart from any extra

---

[169] Buchholz introduced the use of antibiotic-loaded cement in 1970. Buchholz and Engelbrecht (1970); Wahlig and Buchholz (1972); Wahlig *et al.* (1984); Taggart *et al.* (2002).

dynamic component.[170] It is extraordinary. But somebody standing with their hip at 90°, the inward force on that hip is beyond belief. I cannot believe that there will not be a need for revision in the future.

I came on to the scene at a time of operating, relatively speaking. I had the benefits of the English trio: Ring, Charnley and McKee. They had all the ingredients, albeit with different materials and the like, except for titanium and for HAC [hydroxyapatite coating].[171] When the hip escaped from this country, it was largely the polyethylene against polished metal that was the popular image, and once it was released, especially in the US, because of the crude method of operating, without even the instruction that people [surgeons] would get from Wrightington, there was a vast failure rate. But it was also happening in this country, proportionally the same, I suspect. Alongside this, there was a lot of development activity on the Continent, although we live next door to them, remarkably we know nothing about [their work]. Now, if we forget

---

[170] Professor John Paul wrote: 'The Biomechanics Group at the University of Strathclyde was asked by Mr James Tulloch Brown FRCS to assist in the design of a device for fixation of femoral neck fractures. A review of the literature provided the value of hip joint force of 2.4 times body weight when standing on one leg [Inman (1947); Pauwels (1935)] and the inter-segment forces and moments at the hip during level walking [Bresler and Frankel (1950)], but no values of joint force in walking had been established. We set up a gait laboratory, manufacturing a force platform for ground-to-foot force measurement and arranging two 16mm cine cameras viewing from the front and the side of the test subjects, which allowed determination of the three-dimensional coordinates defining the position of the pelvis. This allowed us to calculate the inter-segment force and moments acting between the thigh and the pelvis. Values of forces in the relevant muscles were calculated by selections from the two groups of extensor muscles, two groups of flexors and one group for abductors and one for adductors. The joint force was then calculated from the ground force and the relevant muscle forces at time intervals of 0.02 seconds. The calculated joint force values were from 2 to 9 times body weight (a mean of 4.53). The 9 times value was developed by one subject walking at 2 m/s [metres/second] with a stride length of 2.2m. These studies suggest that the hip joint force in walking depends largely on the product of body weight and stride length. Joint forces of 6.6 and 5.8 times body weight respectively were found, and entry or leaving a car at 5.3 times. Mr Reg Elson [page 83] must be extrapolating from the foregoing data since we have not undertaken tests on runners. Tests undertaken on two of the patients who had received the telemetering hip joint replacement developed by Bergmann *et al.* [(1993)] gave curves of variation with time similar to those calculated from gait analysis although the maximum values differed by approximately 16 per cent on average. An important feature of hip joint loading is the direction of the joint force relative to the axis of the femur. In walking, this may be 35 degrees in the frontal plane and 15 degrees in the sagittal plane. The latter gives rise to a strong twisting moment between a femoral implant and the shaft of the femur and the effect will be greater in stair negotiation and sprinting.' E-mail to Mrs Lois Reynolds, 29 October 2006. See Paul (1966, 1999, 2005); Markolf *et al.* (1979); Berme and Paul (1979); Stansfield *et al.* (2003). See also van den Bogert *et al.* (1999).

[171] Stephenson *et al.* (1991).

infection, which is one source of loosening (I will return to this later, if there's time), the main serious problem is one of mechanical loosening – instability, dislocation and impingement – something that is obvious quickly. Mechanical loosening, so-called, is due to osteolysis, due to whatever cause – and that can be a bad surgeon, as has been shown in the Trent Regional Arthroplasty panel.[172] Otherwise it can simply be due to polyethylene debris. Now Michael Freeman was pivotal in my development in this train of thought, at an illustrious meeting in Paris that shall be nameless, I think, 20 years ago. Michael gave a lecture, which was unique in my experience, because he produced one slide which was a failed, cemented prosthesis, with all the characteristic fluffiness and in the radiolucent zones.[173] He then challenged the audience to say what could be done to revise this. Dutifully, because I was a cementer, I put my hand up and said, 'I would cement it'. Subsequently, after that brilliant presentation, which you [Michael Freeman] don't remember, but which changed my view, to the fact that revision surgery almost certainly should entail uncemented components, unless you are dealing with some impossible situation with very, very thin weak bone, or perhaps a stove-type femur, or perhaps an acetabulum that's gone right through. Forgetting infection, I think that non-cemented revision is probably going to be the answer. I feel sad about it, because I have always been a cementer, but I must confess that if I were beginning again, I would be an un-cementer. I would still want to have cement available, and I would still want to know how to use it, because it is a very special tool, that has, I think, a special place.

I want to pay tribute to Hans Buchholz, a name that has been mentioned. Buchholz produced a most remarkable series of joint replacements, the principles of which have survived, but he also introduced this naive concept of throwing some antibiotics into the cement and it would give you protection. There is no doubt that it does. Whether that's a good thing, or whether we should be purists and rely on prophylactic antibiotics or clean air or both preferably, is not part of the argument. I think I will finish by just saying that failure is terribly important, it's very important that we have revisions, because if you don't have revisions, you wouldn't really know which was the best prosthesis to use, would you?[174]

Lettin: Before you finish in terms of revision, may I ask when the concept of immediate replacement began in this period that we are considering? Initially

---

[172] The Trent register was established in 1990. Harper *et al.* (1998); Fender *et al.* (2000); Hassan *et al.* (2000).

[173] A radiolucent zone in an X-ray permits the passage of X-rays, unlike one that is radio-opaque.

[174] See Table 1, page 75.

you did nothing, you basically left it [**From the floor:** Are you talking about infection?] [Yes], with an excision arthroplasty.

Elson: Until Buchholz introduced the one-stage – and sometimes two-stage – replacement with antibiotic-loaded cement, the majority of Charnley's cases were always converted to a pseudoarthrosis, which was the only thing that could be done. I was privileged to treat some of John Charnley's infections; there were very, very few, as you might imagine, and he didn't believe in the Buchholz technique at first.[175]

Lettin: It went against the accepted normal surgical principle didn't it, to put foreign material into an infected area.

Elson: Absolutely, but there is no question that it works and it protects, for example, in morselized grafting, if you choose to go down that line.

Lettin: What was the date of that? When did we start?

Elson: As far as I am concerned, 1978.

Lettin: That was what I wanted to get down, because this was rather a big thing wasn't it.

Elson: I thought it was, and I did some animal studies in this country and checked the various things that Buchholz recommended and it all seemed to fit together.[176] I remember Buchholz putting his hand on my shoulder and saying, 'Elson, you will come and work for me in Germany', and I said, 'Not on your nelly'. Anyway I went to Germany for a year – Buchholz had his faults – there's no question – but he had charisma.

I will tell you one little story. Buchholz came across just after the war, met Charnley, who wouldn't talk to him because he had a sabre scar on his face. Charnley sent him away again, but Buchholz came back and by that time we were in the RCH 1000 high-density polyethylene era [1965]. Buchholz asked Charnley, 'What is this stuff?' He had already been to see Maurice Müller, and Maurice had got the magic formula from Charnley. Müller said, 'Oh, it's a trade secret' and wouldn't tell him. Charnley said to Buchholz: 'The stuff was made in your country, you might as well use it, mightn't you?'

---

[175] See note 169.

[176] Elson *et al.* (1977a and b).

Lettin: I think you haven't told us your contribution to this, but perhaps John Read, who was also a reviser, will tell us about these early revision techniques?

Read: The earliest revision technique was taking everything out and trying to cure the infection, and then often leaving them as a Girdlestone.[177] Later we started revising them, and with antibiotic-loaded cement.

Lettin: Ian Stephen has gone, I think, because he would probably, well, Robin Ling would have a lot to say on the subject of putting bone grafts in and other things into infected surgical beds.[178]

Elson: Alan, I think we should distinguish between revision for sterile loosening and for infection, they are two different things, except that in both the endosteal surface of the femur is damaged; very quickly it becomes smooth and glass-like and slimey, and is totally unsuited for cementing.[179] I spent hours and hours and hours trying to cut grooves to give some key, but however carefully you do it, you cannot mimic the virgin rugose endosteal surface. Once the failure is recognized to be sufficiently progressive, revision should be done as soon as possible.

Lettin: I think we will have to press on. Has anybody anything else to say? Keith.

Tucker: We haven't mentioned anaesthetists and anaesthetics. I wonder if we could, just for a moment, because they are quite important from the historical perspective. I remember how worried we were when cement was introduced to the femoral canal, when, with pressurization, occasionally patients could die.[180] The anaesthetists at that time tried to get the blood pressure up because they were worried about it falling, something of a reverse from today's practice. Hip surgery has promoted specialist anaesthetists who now understand the use of spinal anaesthetics, epidurals, etc., and this has made hip replacement a lot safer. In the late 1960s and through the 1970s most patients had three units of blood as a minimum for a hip replacement, but with the advances of anaesthesia and the better understanding of haemodynamics, nowadays, many patients don't have a transfusion.

---

[177] See note 5.

[178] Halliday *et al.* (2003).

[179] See note 168.

[180] Phillips *et al.* (1971, 1973); Buerkle and Eftekhar (1975); Oh *et al.* (1978); Randall *et al.* (2006).

Lettin: Yes, most of you probably remember that Hugh Phillips and I and my anaesthetist published a paper in the *British Medical Journal* (*BMJ*) – only the second one I ever had in the *BMJ* – and that was on the cardiovascular effects of implanted acrylic cement.[181] This fits in with what I was saying earlier about this chap at North Hill Plastics,[182] because he paid for a technician, but I am not going to go into that any further. It was something that concerned the DoH, which set up a working party on it, because people were getting alarmed about patients dying while having mainly cemented Thompson's prostheses for fractures, rather than THR. We won't pursue that, but you are quite right that the advances in anaesthetics are very important.

We are getting close to time and we ought just to talk about the results of follow-up, and we have heard how difficult it is and how we haven't done our job properly, but Michael Wroblewski certainly has. I beg your pardon, Graham.

Deane: Sorry, I didn't manage to catch your eye, Chairman, on a point on anaesthetics. When I was in Oxford, this business of drop in blood pressure associated with cement was being looked into. They came to the conclusion – I am a little bit hazy on this, not knowing the anaesthetic side – that the use of a neuroleptic-analgesic type of general anaesthetic seemed to avoid this particular problem.

Another aside as well, there was another particular anaesthetic problem with the airway in juvenile rheumatoids. Malcolm Swann knows better than I do, and along with my predecessor George Arden, that operating on juvenile rheumatoids' hips in the days before the laryngeal mask was hazardous, due to the dreadful airway they so often had that prevented intubation. The anaesthetists used a clever drug called ketamine. Now, the side effect of ketamine, from the surgeon's point of view, is that everything can bleed profusely, making control of the bleeding difficult. I am sure Malcolm Swann will probably add to this, that ketamine added to the difficulties of surgery already complicated by the distorted anatomy of these children. However, ketamine made it possible to perform surgery safely. It has now gone out of use with the development of newer techniques such as the laryngeal mask that can deal with the difficult airway and has made a lot of difference to this aspect.[183]

---

[181] Phillips *et al.* (1971); Charnley (1970); Ring (1970a).

[182] See note 123.

[183] D'Arcy *et al.* (1976).

Lettin: Am I right in thinking that at Norwich you have a pretty comprehensive follow-up of McKee's replacements? Who's going to answer that, Keith or your follow-up lady Clare Darrah?

Tucker: In 2005 the British Hip Society invited practitioners who work with hip surgeons to come to our annual scientific meeting. It was recognized that there were many people up and down the country helping with the evaluation of hip replacements and the management of patients post-operatively. After the meeting, the Arthroplasty Care Practitioners Association was born, through the efforts of Clare Darrah here and her colleagues.[184] Thus, through hip replacement another step forward has been made in the care and long-term follow-up of hip replacements.

Darrah: For those of you who don't know, I have been employed at Norwich for the last ten years and been involved in what we call our joint replacement follow-up programme, so we are keeping an eye on all of our implants in Norwich, some of them very historical, and some are more recent. We have just founded the Arthroplasty Care Practitioners Association, who are mainly physiotherapists and nurses working with orthopaedic surgeons around the country, collecting data, so I hope that the tide has turned and that with the National Joint Register doing its bit as well, that we are actually going to have better outcome data in the next ten or 15 years.

Lettin: What about McKee's early results? Michael Wroblewski can go back to Charnley's results, with almost continuous records from the beginning, as I understand it. Can you do that with McKee or not? [**Tucker:** No.] We can't really have a comparison of the long-term results from metal-on-metal, and the metal-on-plastic.[185]

Heywood-Waddington: Chairman, as part of my preparation for this meeting, I reviewed my own 'audit', as I like to call it, of the early McKee replacements to compare them with each other and with my own, while I still did these operations. I also tried to take account of any modifications introduced. I

---

[184] Clare Darrah (Norwich), Jill Pope (Liverpool), Justine Greaves (Clydebank), Cathy Jenkins (Oxford), Judith Learmont and Morag Trayner (Edinburgh), Lindsay Smith (Weston-super-Mare), Barbara Selvon (Sheffield), together with Malcolm Binns and Gordon Bannister were involved in this initiative. For background details, see www.britishhipsociety.com/Newsletter%20Sept%202005.doc (visited 1 August 2006).

[185] Wilson *et al.* (1972); Patterson and Brown (1972).

obtained information formally, and was privy to those minuted at the meeting in Austria every year, until about 1979, 1980.[186] Among these were papers by McKee himself, giving his 10-year and 12-year follow-ups of his own hips,[187] and by Christopher Partridge from Worthing. There was also a paper by Dandy and Theodorou, comprising a restrospective review of 1042 McKee hip replacements, performed in Norwich between 1965–72. One in 12 of these required revision at some stage.[188] I also entered into informal correspondence with colleagues I knew to be performing this operation.

From all this evidence I came to the conclusion that the overall results were remarkably similar, irrespective of whether the surgeons concerned had received formal training in Norwich, or not, and independently of any minor modification to the technique that they may have introduced, and irrespective of the 'learning curve'. There was about 85 per cent to 90 per cent patient satisfaction rate up to five years and an ultimate 10 per cent to 15 per cent revision rate overall. As one would expect, most of the early revisions were due to surgical error rather than inherent defect.

Wroblewski: When we talk about long-term results, and long not being defined, there is one thing that I don't think that anybody – I don't only mean here, but anywhere – has actually realized that long-term results can only be achieved in young patients. So, when we talk about long-term results, they are results in young patients. Let me give you a bit of information, if I may. If we assume that all the patients are operated on day one as we do for survivorship analysis,[189] for every year of follow-up, the mean age of patients at primary surgery, those that are still attending, declines by eight months. So to get a 25-year follow-up, that patient at the time of surgery must have been about 50. So it is not just long-term results, but long-term results in young patients. So when we hear that a new design or material, especially metal-on-metal, is suitable for young patients, the question is: 'Have you got long-term follow-up?' Long-term follow-ups are results in young patients.

---

[186] See note 95.

[187] McKee (1974, 1982); McKee and Chen (1973).

[188] Dandy and Theodorou (1975). A retrospective review of 1042 McKee–Farrar prostheses inserted in Norwich from January 1965 to December 1972.

[189] For Charnley survivorship analysis, see Wroblewski *et al.* (2002); for the Stanmore, see Dobbs (1980). Survivorship was determined from modified life tables according to Armitage (1971): 408–14.

Lettin: What about your follow-ups of the early Charnley replacements?

Wroblewski: Those that are alive? You see, originally the patients' mean age was 65, and that has basically remained unchanged. We have early results. The longest follow-up we at Wrightington have is 42 years and going strong.[190]

Lettin: But in terms of the proportions of those early ones?

Wroblewski: It is age, how old those patients were at the time of surgery.

Lettin: But in terms of the survival analysis which takes that into consideration, as you have already said, how does that compare with McKee?

Wroblewski: I don't know what the McKee results are, but if we look at patients with rheumatoid arthritis, a mean age of 36 years at the time of surgery, and all under the age of 51 by the 32-year follow-up, the patient dies before revision becomes indicated, the arthroplasty outlasts the patient.[191]

Tucker: I want to point out, for the historical record, that today's meeting has reinforced and added to what has been happening over the past 30 years. Hip surgeons have been dedicated to keeping records and everything we have been talking about today bears witness to this. Out of hip replacement has come the *Journal of Arthroplasty*, which Mike Freeman has run so well [as European Editor, 1996 to 2001],[192] and endless articles in the *JBJS* (*Journal of Bone and Joint Surgery*).[193] This is part of our history, but it has stimulated orthopaedic surgeons to look even more critically at what they do and continue to do.

Lettin: I am going to ask Peter Ring if he would like the last word. He almost had the first one, and hasn't really said a great deal, although he has lived through all of this. What about your own results, Peter?

Ring: The results which I have had fall into two groups. If you use uncemented metal-on-metal implants, you can get a 20-year survivorship of 95 per cent. If you use uncemented metal-on-plastic, it's much less good. I don't know what

---

[190] See note 21.

[191] Professor Mike Wroblewski wrote: 'With survivorship analysis the end point can be taken either as revision or the patient's death. In young patients with rheumatoid arthritis, "end point revision" gives higher survivorship than "end point death".' Note on draft transcript, 24 October 2006.

[192] Hungerford (2005).

[193] The *JBJS* has been published as separate American and British journals since 1948, distinguished by the appropriate mark, (A) or (B).

20 years is, but even at 10 to 12 years, you are looking at 10 to 12 per cent of failures, and the difference between the two is clearly the effect of polyethylene debris upon the interface both on the outside of the cup and on the femoral side. Of the metal-on-metal debris, which we have seen, there have been three or four examples of aggregates of metal forming cysts near the joint, but that is no more than three or four in some 1200 patients.[194] We have looked at the interface between the implant and bone in loosening implants, and certainly you get metal debris down there, but you do not seem to get a reaction at that point. So there may be some problems with the long-term effects of metal, but the survivorship does look quite good.

The other thing that strikes me, having listened to this, is that I operated for most of my time within a theatre that was also used by a gynaecological team and occasionally for a general surgical emergency. We used a horizontal laminar air flow system,[195] no exhausts or anything like that, and the advantage of your horizontal system is that you can sterilize all your implements and apart from the implants, you have got everything ready there, everything for the actual replacement, everything for breaking the femur when you put the implant in too tightly, and that has a great advantage, and it seemed to us to be better than the vertical system. And as far as infection was concerned, we were able to do 1000 metal-on-metal implants without anything other than superficial infection.[196] So I think when people talk about the infection rate in total hip replacement, it's got to be associated with the statement that these are implants that are cemented into position, and I do think there is a difference. Most people with uncemented implants don't look upon infection as a major problem.[197]

Sweetnam: May I just briefly ask one question. All of us here have the accumulated experience of witnessing the development of hip surgery. We have lived through a most exciting time in surgery, and, in fact, I think we have been discussing one of the greatest advances in surgery ever. We have made some mistakes along the way, I am sure, and I just wonder whether there is any view that we ought to give to those people who may be reading this in many years'

---

[194] Godsiff *et al.* (1992). See also Fitzpatrick *et al.* (1998). This review found the most favourable prostheses in terms of revision rates, at that time, were the Exeter, the Lubinus IP, a German prosthesis, and the Charnley.

[195] Salvati *et al.* (1982).

[196] Ring (1974).

[197] Ring (1978, 1981, 1983); Bertin *et al.* (1985).

time, as to how those mistakes might be avoided in the future and particularly what the mistakes were. I think it's quite important, looking back over 30 years of a new surgical procedure, to note that it was a triumph in the end for the vast majority of patients, but a failure for some less fortunate, who were in receipt of less than perfect prostheses.[198]

Lettin: I have tried to get people to say what they think were the causes of hip failure, and I didn't really have a great deal of success in pinning down people as to whether it was technical. I think John Older probably summed it all up by saying that it was a mixture of all these things. I don't know whether you feel that you can do any better.

Sweetnam: I only asked the question because I knew the answer. The answer is that we have failed miserably in surveillance. I mean we have been watching a new procedure develop over 35, maybe 40 years, and we are still asking questions that we can't answer because we do not have the correct surveillance procedures in place and I think personally that's the message for the future.

Freeman: May I add something to that? I totally agree, and although there is no convincing evidence, I don't think that new implants are any better. So it may be true that we are moving forwards, but I am not sure that we have evidence that we are moving forwards, since the opening period that you described, Chairman.

Mr Michael Wilson: Could I just say I am extremely happy to be here today in this august company and one of the things that my father ['Ginger' Wilson] was very keen on, was to take notes, meticulous notes, and we have a cellar full of patients' records, which he referred to occasionally if anyone rang up. He could find them within about a matter of minutes, through an extraordinary cross-filing index that I never really understood myself. But that was one of his great things, that things should be written down and noted particularly. The other thing was that, I think, part of the reason that John Scales dealt exclusively with

---

[198] For example, in 1998 the DoH issued a Hazard Warning Notice [HN9801] due to 'poor short-term performance of the femoral component' to hospitals to recall and review all patients who received a 3-M™ Capital™ Hip implant between 1991–97, when the device was discontinued, less than 2 per cent of UK hip replacement operations over that period. A fund established by 3M Healthcare paid for clinical review and revision if needed, for these patients, which closed in 2003, leaving further care to the NHS. See www.dh.gov.uk/PublicationsAndStatistics/PressReleases/PressReleasesNotices/fs/en?CONTENT_ID=4024446&chk=AMG%2BAI; and www.dh.gov.uk/assetRoot/04/01/49/75/04014975.pdf (visited 14 November 2006). National Audit Office (2000).

Phyllis' company, was that they wanted to cut down on any variables so that the quality of the materials they received wasn't in question and obviously that helps with the analysis of data later on.

Lettin: I think we have to bring things to a conclusion.

Dowson: The discussion brings to mind one of Winston Churchill's observations:[199] 'Success is never final'.

Lettin: Thank you very much, everyone, for keeping very much to time and I hope that the Wellcome Trust's History of Twentieth Century Medicine Group have what they wanted. We have drifted away from history, I am afraid, and come up to the present time, but there we are, that's the way it went. You wanted a free and easy discussion.

Christie: Absolutely. I want to thank you all for participating in this afternoon's seminar and also to thank Alan Lettin for his excellent chairing of this occasion.

---

[199] Enright (ed.) (2001): 92.

Appendix 1

Notes on Materials by Professor Alan Swanson[200]

Metallic Alloys

Corrosion-resisting steel (stainless steel)	Iron (Fe) plus a small percentage of carbon (C) and about 20 per cent chromium (Cr) and 10 per cent nickel (Ni). Driven largely by the needs of joint replacement, both the composition and the manufacture of the surgical grades have been refined until they are now very different from the general-purpose alloys from which they are derived, with many other constituents to improve resistance to fatigue and corrosion. Its strength varies according to whether it is annealed or coldworked.
Cobalt–chromium alloys	Cobalt (Co) with a substantial percentage of chromium (Cr) and smaller quantities of other elements. Highly resistant to wear and corrosion (for example, as hard facings in earth-moving machinery) and used by dentists because of their suitability for precision-investment casting and their corrosion resistance. Fifty years ago, and probably is still, the only alloy type that can be seriously considered for both surfaces of one bearing. Nobody has yet produced or discovered another material, or if they have, it is impossibly expensive.
Titanium alloys	Titanium (Ti) is lighter than steel or cobalt and has good corrosion resistance, but it and its alloys were very expensive 50 years ago and very difficult to manufacture. Titanium alloys retain their strength and stiffness to higher temperatures than do aluminium alloys, so they are used for aircraft that fly fast enough (significantly supersonic) to undergo significant kinetic heating. The needs of the aerospace industry had led to development which made it practical, and an alloy with some aluminium and vanadium in it was being used for femoral prostheses by 1978. The Standard was revised and republished in 1996.

---

[200] Additional information provided by Mr Ravi Kunzru and Mr Victor Wheble.

Polymers

Polymethylmethacrylate
(PMMA)
(Perspex®, Plexiglass®)

Used as a solid material by the Judet brothers for femoral heads [Judet and Judet (1950), see also Appendix 3], but has been a major factor in hip replacement since c. 1960.
Used as the monomer, with an accelerator, and inserted between prosthesis and bone and allowed to polymerize in situ, it takes about 10 minutes to form bone cement.
Two proprietary brands of PMMA were used in the UK: CMW and Simplex [North Hill Plastics], essentially the same chemically, but different in detail. Charnley used CMW. See note 9.

Polytetrafluorethylene (PTFE)
(Fluon®, Teflon®)

Low friction, but not particularly wear-resistant. See Figure 4.

Polyethylene
(UHMWPE, HDP)

Took over from PTFE in 1961 as the material of choice for the plastic element of a metal-on-plastic bearing in hip replacement. Friction is higher than with PTFE, but still much lower than metal-on-metal, and the mechanical properties are better, leading to better wear resistance. Widely used outside orthopaedics, but the needs of joint replacement have driven developments to obtain better wear performance, particularly by increasing the length of the molecular chains to give ultra-high molecular weight and high-density versions. As with all polymers, the additives that are usual for non-surgical purposes (fillers, colours, lubricants) must be strictly controlled or eliminated.

Ceramics

Alumina
(aluminium oxide)

Like most metallic oxides, this ceramic is hard and capable of being finished to a very high polish with suitable machinery. It is found in less-refined forms in general engineering where its brittleness is acceptable, but the orthopaedic form is less brittle and more homogeneous, permitting better surface finish and lower wear rates.

Zirconia
(zirconium oxide)

One of many other ceramics that are potentially useful to orthopaedics and has been used as an alloying constituent with alumina.

Appendix 2

Surgical implant material standards, 1960–70s
by Mr Victor Wheble (28 June 2006)

There were a few British standards available for materials used in making prostheses in 1960–70 and standardization work was just beginning in this field, possibly also in other countries.[201] There were no generally accepted International Standards at that time. The British Standard for wrought stainless steel (BS3531) was only made redundant when suitable International Standards were finally developed. The first group of these were published in 1970 and included stainless steels and chrome–cobalt alloys, followed by titanium and titanium alloys in 1979, though work at the international level on many of the other metallic materials had commenced in 1972. At the beginning it was a bit of a 'free for all', though the British were working towards standardization of other materials, and there was standardization activity in France, Germany, Switzerland and the USA. New materials were being suggested from time to time, but they were not always accepted for Standardization.

The inaugural meeting of the ISO Technical Committee [ISO/TC150] took place in London in 1972, and a start was made at a meeting in Pforzheim, Germany, in the following year. At the second meeting in Copenhagen, Sweden, in 1975, discussion took place on the standardization of such matters as materials for implants. A task group at that conference was set up to look at quality control as this was the beginning of the system of making international standards for bone and joint replacements. The large number of relevant ISO standards that subsequently appeared has been increased further as a result of the European Union (EU) setting up their CEN standards organization. Most of the CEN standards are the same, in essence, as those produced by ISO, because they are generally written by the same delegates. The only serious difference between ISO and CEN standards is the legal requirement for compliance with CEN standards throughout the EU. ISO standards are not legally binding in all the world, but they are accepted in most of the countries involved in implant manufacture, and companies who make implants do have to be careful how they produce their products. Such standards are not as rigid as they would be

---

[201] Scales (1965) describes the early work of the British Standards Committee, SGC/18, under the chairmanship of Mr Norman Capener, and the creation of BS3531:1962, the basic requirements for metal surgical implants, twist drills and screwdrivers. See also Capener (1965); British Standards Institution (1962, 1964). BS3531-1 covered stainless steel; and BS3531-2 cobalt-chromium alloys.

if they were legally binding, but perhaps they do constitute the best available method of quality control that is acceptable by manufacturers on a worldwide basis. I must emphasize, however, that the CEN standards do have legal status in the EU.

I have no record of other relevant British Standard numbers before 1978, but there were many heated discussions in the BSI and ISO meetings on the subject of materials between 1967 and 1978. Materials supplied to manufacturers in England during the 1970s would have been made to such British Standards as existed. I doubt whether there were British Standards on other materials than stainless steel. It is more likely that various formulae for chrome–cobalt alloys were being used by different manufacturers and probably the same situation applied with other materials, like titanium and the titanium alloys. (The 'DIS' in the standards numbering system means a Draft International Standard that is not yet fully approved.)

All International Standards are brought to attention every five years and if necessary they are then revised, but more often are accepted for a further five-year period. ASTM Standards are American in origin and are also revised in the same way. Some of these eventually become ISO Standards after revision.

The International Organization for Standardization (ISO) produces Standards for metallic materials that are generally acceptable worldwide.[202] If there is a need to quote the compositions of these materials, the details can be obtained from the ISO Central Secretariat at 1 Rue de Varembe, Case postale 56, CH-1211 Genève 20, Switzerland (Tel +41 22 749 01 11, or the Sales Department +41 22 734 10 79); catalogue available at www.iso.org/iso/en/CatalogueListPage. CatalogueList (visited 11 July 2006).

---

[202] See, for example, BS EN 12010:1998. Non-active surgical implants, joint replacement implants, particular requirements. The international equivalent is EN 12010:1998, which covers implants (surgical), joints (anatomy), orthopaedic equipment, prosthetic devices, performance, life (durability), surface texture, marking, inspection, sterilization (hygiene), instructions for use, compatibility, metals, alloys, non-metals, and medical equipment. Standards that apply are: ISO/5832-1:1997; ISO/5832-2:1993; ISO/5832-3:1996; ISO/5832-4:1996; ISO/5832-5:1993; ISO/5832-6:1997; ISO/5832-7:1994; ISO/5832-8:1997; ISO/5832-9:1995; ISO/5832-10:1996; ISO/5832-11:1994; ISO/5832-12:1996; ISO/5833:1992; ISO/5834-1:1997; ISO/5834-2:1997; ISO/6474:1994; ISO/13356; ISO/5839:1985; ISO/6018:1987; ISO/7206-1:1995; ISO/7206-4:1989; ISO/7206-5:1992; ISO/7206-6:1992; ISO/7206-8:1995; ISO/7206-9:1994; ISO/7207-1:1994; ISO/DIS 7207-2:1996; ISO/8828:1988; ISO/TR 9325:1989; ISO/TR 9326:1989; ISO/9583:1993; ISO/9584:1993; BS6324-1; BS6324-2; BS6324-3; BS6324-4; BS6324-5; ASTM F 746; ASTM F 897; ASTM F 1147; ASTM F 1223; ASTM F 370; ASTM F 604; ASTM F 997; ASTM F 1185; ASTM F 1351; ASTM F 1378; NF S 94-065; 93/42/EEC; EN ISO/14630:1997; ISO/7206-2:1996; ISO/14630:1997.

Relevant standards for surgical implants during the period 1970–96

(a) Metallic materials

Part 1: Wrought stainless steel British Standard, BS 3531:1968.	ISO/DIS 5832–1. (1970)
Part 2: Unalloyed titanium Revised 1993.	ISO/5832–2. (1978)
Part 3: Wrought titanium-6-aluminium 4-vanadium alloy Revised, 1980, 1996.	ISO/5832–3. (1978)
Part 4: Cobalt–chromium–molybdenum casting alloy Revised, 1996.	ISO/5832–4. (1978)
Part 5: Wrought cobalt–chromium–tungsten–nickel alloy Revised, 1993, 1997.	ISO/5832–5. (1980)
Part 6: Wrought cobalt–nickel–chromium–molybdenum alloy Revised, 1997.	ISO/5832–6. (1980)
Part 7: Forgeable and cold-formed cobalt–chromium–nickel molybdenum–iron alloy	ISO/5832–7. (1994)
Part 8: Wrought cobalt–nickel–chromium–molybdenum–tungsten–iron alloy. Revised, 1997.	ISO/5832–8. (1987)
Part 9: Wrought high nitrogen stainless steel Revised, 1995.	ISO/5832–9. (1992)
Part 10: Wrought titanium 5-aluminium 2.5–iron alloy Revised, 1996.	ISO/5832–10. (1993)
Part 11: Wrought titanium 6-aluminium 7-niobium alloy	ISO/5832–11: (1994)
Part 12: Wrought cobalt–chromium–molybdenum alloy	ISO/5832–12: (1997)

(b) Other materials

Implants for surgery – acrylic resin cements	ISO/5833: (1992)
Ultra-high Molecular Weight Polyethylene (UHMWPE): Part 1: Powder form	ISO/5834–1: (1985)
Ultra-high Molecular Weight Polyethylene (UHMWPE): Part 2: Moulded form	ISO/5834–2: (1995)

For example, composition of selected standards:

Element	Standards		
	ISO/5832-5 (1993) Co-Cr-Ni-W (%)	ISO/5832-6 (1997) Co-Cr-Mo (%)	ISO/5832-7 (1994) Co-Cr-Ni-Mo-Fe (%)
carbon (C)	0.05	0.25	0.15
chromium (Cr)	20.0	27.0	2.0
cobalt (Co)	50.25	61.5	40.85
iron (Fe)	2.5	0.75	15.0
manganese (Mn)	1.0	1.0	2.0
molybdenum (Mo)	0.0	6.0	7.0
nickel (Ni)	10.0	2.5	15.0
silicon (Si)	1.0	1.0	0.0
tungsten (W)	15.2	0.0	0.0

Appendix 3

Selected prosthetic hips[203]

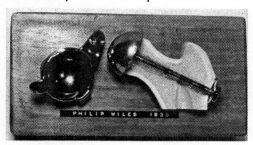
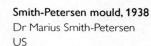

Wiles' acetabular cup and resurface of head of the femur, 1938
Mr Philip Wiles
The London Hospital, UK

Single bolt-on femoral component, stainless steel, 1938.

See: Wiles (1958).
See also Figure 3.

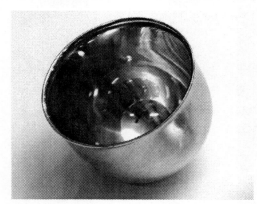

Smith-Petersen mould, 1938
Dr Marius Smith-Petersen
US

Vitallium® mould (cobalt–chromium–molybdenum alloy) arthroplasty interposed between refashioned surfaces of acetabulum and head of the femur.

See: Smith-Petersen (1939).
Also appears as Figure 11.

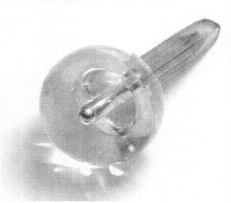

Judet brothers' acrylic femur head-replacement, late 1940s
Drs Jean and Robert Judet
France

Acrylic, short-stem, mushroom shape 'resection-reconstruction' of the femur head, with stem designed to pass through to the neck of the femur.

See: Judet and Judet (1950);
An advertisement from 1950 is reproduced in Tennent and Eastwood (1998): 386.

---

[203] For advertisements of various prostheses available, for example in 1973, see www.jbjs.org.uk/cgi/issue_pdf/backmatter_pdf/55-B/3.pdf (visited 12 December 2006).

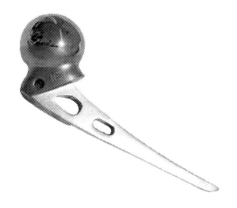

Moore intramedullary endoprosthesis, 1950s –
Dr Austin Moore
US

Later model of Moore Vitallium® prosthesis, tapered stem and collar, uncemented.

See: Moore and Bohlman (1943).

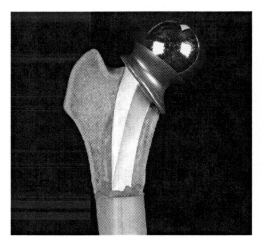

Thompson intramedullary prosthesis, 1953 –
Dr Frederick Thompson
US

Curved solid Vitallium® stem, large head, cemented. Introduced in the US in 1953.

See: Thompson (1952).

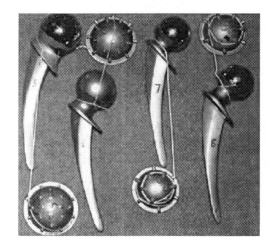

McKee total hip replacement, 1956 –
Mr Kenneth McKee
Norfolk and Norwich Hospital, UK

Vitallium® prosthesis with various cup models from 1963.

Manufactured by: Down Brothers Ltd, London; later Hunton Engineering, Norwich.

See: McKee (1951);
McKee and Watson-Farrar (1966).
See also Figures 6 and 7.

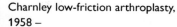

Charnley low-friction arthroplasty, 1958 –

Sir John Charnley
Wrightington Hospital, nr Wigan, UK

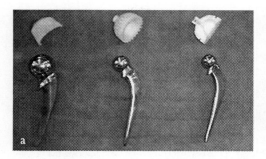

(a) L to R: Thompson prosthesis with a PTFE cup; Low-frictional torque, 28mm diameter femoral head and PTFE cup with maximum external diameter; 25mm diameter femoral head with PTFE cup.

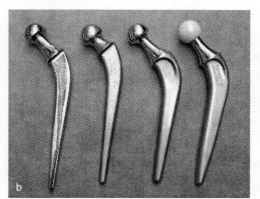

(b) L to R: 4 models, 1962–86: original 1962 flat-back 316J stainless steel stem with a polished finish; 1974, round-back Charnley stem with a vaquasheen finish; 1975, round-back Charnley stem with a flange; 1986, Charnley stem (Ortron 90) and Alumina Ceramic head.

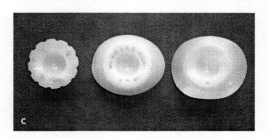

(c) L to R: 1962, original Charnley cup; 1977, pressure injection flange added to the cup to improve acetabular fixation; 1982, Ogee flange added to the cup to stabilize acetabular fixation by enhancing cement pressurization.

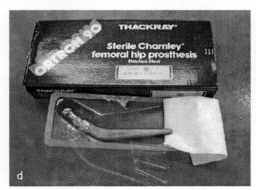

(d) The Ortron 90, 1980.

Manufactured by: Thackray, 1962–90; DuPuy, from 1990.

See: Charnley (1960, 1961).
See also Figures 4 and 15.

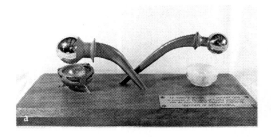

Stanmore total hip replacement, 1963 –
Mr John Scales
Institute of Orthopaedics, RNOH,
Stanmore, UK

(a) L to R: 1963–72: Mark 1–5, cobalt–chrome-on-cobalt–chrome stem and cup; 1970s cobalt–chrome-on-plastic stem and cup.

(b) Stanmore range with various diameter heads and femoral components of various lengths, c. 1970s.

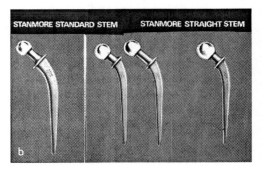

(c) Stanmore ceramic head, Alivium (a vacuum cast cobalt base alloy) stem and polyethylene cups, c. 1970s.

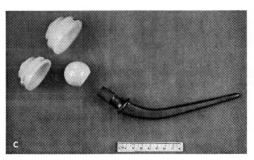

(d) Stanmore: 3 matt stems: bottom to top: Mk10 32mm head, Alivium, standard stem, c. mid-1960s; Biomet 29mm head, straight stem, c. mid-1970s; Alivium stem, 29mm head, c. mid-1970s.

Manufactured by: Zimmer Orthopaedic Ltd to 1984; Biomet from 1984

See: Duff-Barclay et al. (1966); Scales and Wilson (1969); Wilson and Scales (1973). See also Figure 17.

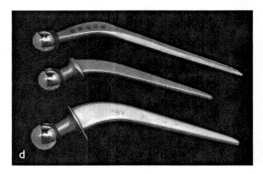

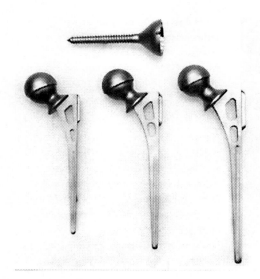

Ring total hip replacement, 1968 –
Mr Peter Ring,
Redhill Group of Hospitals, UK

Uncemented, metal-on-metal implant in cobalt–chrome with single pelvic component and three sizes of femoral stem.
Manufactured by: Downs Surgical Ltd, Mitcham, Surrey.

See: Ring (1968, 1970).
See also Figure 5.

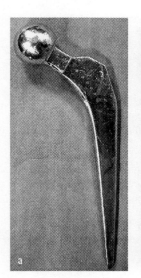
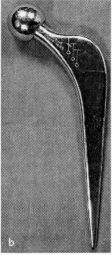

Exeter total hip replacement, 1970 –
Professor Robin Ling
Princess Elizabeth Orthopaedic Hospital, Exeter, UK
Dr Clive Lee
University of Exeter, UK

(a) In clinical practice from autumn 1970 in polished stainless steel (EN58J) with a head size of 29.75mm, cemented with acrylic bone cement and in two sizes (standard and lightweight). The cup was made from high-density polyethylene in three sizes (not illustrated).

(b) Universal Exeter stem, modular polished, 1988–

Manufactured by: London Splint Company (now Stryker Howmedica Osteonics).

See: Lee and Ling (1974); Ling (1997).
See also Figure 20.

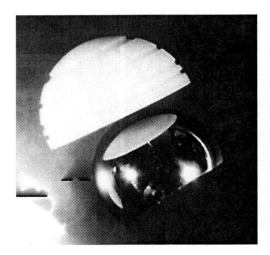

ICLH double cup or resurfacing arthroplasty prosthesis, 1972 –
Professor Michael Freeman
Imperial College and The London Hospital, UK
Professor Alan Swanson
Imperial College, UK

A thinly cemented HDP prosthesis with a stainless steel acetabular cup, first implanted in 1972. A specially designed reamer shaped the femoral head until it fitted into the prosthesis. From 1974 the prosthesis was of cobalt–chrome with an HDP acetabular component.
Left is an X-ray of a bilateral implantation, c. 1980, which is taken from Figure 18.

Manufactured by: Protek AG, Münsingen/ Berne, Switzerland

See: Freeman et al. (1975).
See also Figure 18.

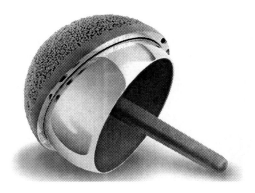

McMinn Birmingham resurfacing, 1991 –
Mr Derek McMinn
Birmingham Nuffield Hospital, Edgbaston, UK

Metal-on-metal prosthesis developed at the Birmingham Nuffield Hospital, and introduced in 1997.

Manufactured by: Midland Medical Technologies Ltd; later Smith & Nephew Bromsgrove Ltd.

See: McMinn et al. (1996).

References

Ahnfelt L, Herberts P, Malchau H, Andersson G B J. (1990) Prognosis of total hip replacement. A Swedish multicenter study of 4664 revisions. *Acta Orthopaedica Scandinavica* **61**: 1–26.

Anderson J. (2006) Greenhouses and body suits: the challenge to knowledge in early hip replacement surgery, 1960–82. In Timmermann C, Anderson J. (eds) *Devices and Designs: Medical technologies in historical perspective.* Houndmills: Palgrave Macmillan, 175–91.

Anderson J, Neary F, Pickstone J V. (forthcoming 2007) *Surgeons, Manufacturers and Patients: A Transatlantic History of the Total Hip Replacement.* Basingstoke: Palgrave.

Anonymous. (1960) Cutting germ risks during operations. *The Times* (30 November): 20.

Anonymous. (1976) The Charnley–Howorth ultra clean air unit. *Nursing Mirror and Midwives Journal* **143**: 58–9.

Anonymous. (1988) Harold Jackson Burrows. *Lives of the Fellows of the Royal College of Surgeons of England* (1974–82) **6**: 56–7.

Ansell B M. (1981) *Chronic Arthritis in Childhood.* Chelmsford: Graves Medical Audiovisual Library [40 slides; original slides seem to have been destroyed in 2006].

Ansell B M, Swann M. (1983) The management of chronic arthritis of children. *Journal of Bone and Joint Surgery (B)* **65**: 536–43.

Ansell B M, Bywaters E G, Spencer P E, Tyler J P. (1997) *Looking Back 1947–85: The Canadian Red Cross Memorial Hospital, Cliveden, Taplow, England.* Buckinghamshire: [privately published by] Barbara M Ansell.

Arden G P, Taylor A R, Ansell B M. (1970) Total hip replacement using the McKee-Farrar prosthesis. In rheumatoid arthritis, Still's disease, and ankylosing spondylitis. *Annals of the Rheumatic Diseases* **29**: 1–5.

Armitage P. (1971) *Statistical Methods in Medical Research.* Oxford: Blackwell.

Barrack R L, Butler R A. (2005) Current status of trochanteric reattachment in complex total hip arthroplasty. *Clinical Orthopaedics and Related Research* **441**: 237–42.

Bechtol C O. (1973) The biomechanics of the epiphyseal lines as a guide to design considerations for the attachment of prosthesis to the musculo-skeletal system. *Journal of Biomedical Materials Research* 7: 343–62.

Benson M K, Goodwin P G, Brostoff J (1975) Metal sensitivity in patients with joint replacement arthroplasties. *British Medical Journal* 4: 374–5.

Berg M, Bergman B R, Hoborn J. (1991) Ultraviolet radiation compared to an ultra-clean air enclosure. Comparison of air bacteria counts in operating rooms. *Journal of Bone and Joint Surgery (B)* **73**: 811–15.

Bergmann G, Graichen F, Rohlmann A. (1993) Hip joint loading during walking and running, measured in two patients. *Journal of Biomechanics* **26**: 969–90.

Berme N, Paul J P. (1979) Load actions transmitted by implants. *Journal of Biomechanical Engineering* **1**: 268–72.

Berntsen A, Bertelsen A. (1952) Preliminary experience with Smith-Petersen's hip cup arthroplasty. *Acta Orthopaedica Scandinavica* **22**: 147–52.

Bertin K C, Freeman M A R, Morscher E, Oeri A, Ring P A. (1985) Cementless acetabular replacement using a pegged polyethylene prosthesis. *Archives of Orthopaedic and Trauma Surgery* **104**: 251–61.

Besong A A, Tipper J L, Ingham E, Stone M H, Wroblewski B M, Fisher J. (1998) Quantitative comparison of wear debris from UHMWPE that has and has not been sterilized by gamma irradiation. *Journal of Bone and Joint Surgery (B)* **80**: 340–4.

Bintcliffe I W. (1983) Effects of using a Charnley–Howorth enclosure in a district general hospital. *Journal of the Royal Society of Medicine* **76**: 262–5.

Black J. (1978) The future of polyethylene. *Journal of Bone and Joint Surgery (B)* **60**: 303–06.

Bloch B. (1958) Bonding of fractures by plastic adhesives; preliminary report. *Journal of Bone and Joint Surgery (B)* **40**: 804–12.

Bloch B, Hastings G W. (1972) *Plastics Materials in Surgery.* 2nd edn. Springfield, IL: Charles C Thomas.

Blowers R, Crew B. (1960). Ventilation of operating theatres. *Journal of Hygiene* **58**: 427–48.

van den Bogert A J, Read L, Nigg B M. (1999) An analysis of hip joint loading during walking, running, and skiing. *Medicine and Science in Sports and Exercise* **31**: 131–42.

Bourdillon R B, Lidwell O M, Thomas J C. (1941) A slit sampler for collecting and counting airborne bacteria. *Journal of Hygiene* **41**: 197–224.

Bourdillon R B, Lidwell O M, Lovelock J E. (1948) *Studies in Air Hygiene*, Medical Research Council, Special Report Series No. 262. London: HMSO.

Bradish C F, Kemp H B, Scales J T, Wilson J N. (1987) Distal femoral replacement by custom-made prostheses. Clinical follow-up and survivorship analysis. *Journal of Bone and Joint Surgery (B)* **69**: 276–84.

Bresler B, Frankel J P. (1950) The forces and moments in the leg during level walking. *Transactions of ASME* **72**: 27–36.

Brigitte M J, Earl R B. (2006) Posterior versus lateral surgical approach for total hip arthroplasty in adults with osteoarthritis. *Cochrane Database Systematic Reviews* **3**: CD003828.

British Standards Institution (BSI). (1962) *BS3531: Metal surgical implants, drills and screwdrivers used for bone surgery*. London: British Standards Institution.

BSI. (1964) *Addendum to BS 3531: Surgical implants of wrought titanium*. London: British Standards Institution.

Brittain H A. (1941) Ischiofemoral arthrodesis. *British Journal of Surgery* **113**: 93–104.

Brittain H A. (1942), *Architectural Principles of Arthrodesis*, Edinburgh: E and S Livingstone Ltd.

Brittain H A. (1948) Ischiofemoral arthrodesis. *Journal of Bone and Joint Surgery (B)* **30**: 642–50.

Buchholz H W, Engelbrecht H. (1970) [Depot effects of various antibiotics mixed with Palacos resins] German. *Der Chirurg: Zeitschrift für alle Gebiete der operativen Medizen* **41**: 511–15.

Buerkle A R Jr, Eftekhar N S. (1975) Fixation of the femoral head prosthesis with methylmethacrylate. *Clinical Orthopaedics and Related Research* **111**: 134–41.

Burrows H J. (1966) Prostheses for arthritic hips. *Journal of Bone and Joint Surgery (B)* **48**: 205–6.

Burrows H J, Wilson J N, Scales J T. (1975) Excision of tumours of humerus and femur, with restoration by internal prostheses. *Journal of Bone and Joint Surgery (B)* **57**: 148–59.

Cameron H U, Freeman M A R. (1977). Surface replacement arthroplasty of the hip. *Journal of Bone and Joint Surgery (B)* **59**: 511–12.

Capener N. (1965) Editorials and annotations: surgical implants. *Journal of Bone and Joint Surgery (B)* **47**: 3–7.

Charnley J. (1950a) *The Closed Treatment of Common Fractures.* Edinburgh: E & S Livingstone. [4th edn, Cambridge: Cambridge University Press, 2005].

Charnley J. (1950b) Method of inserting the Smith-Petersen guide wire. *Journal of Bone and Joint Surgery (B)* **32**: 271–2.

Charnley J. (1953) *Compression Arthrodesis.* Edinburgh: E & S Livingstone.

Charnley J. (1960) Surgery of the hip joint. *British Medical Journal* **i**: 821–6.

Charnley J. (1961) Arthroplasty of the hip – a new operation. *Lancet* **i**: 1, 129.

Charnley J. (1964) The bonding of prostheses to bone by cement. *Journal of Bone and Joint Surgery (B)* **46**: 518–29.

Charnley J. (1965) A biomechanical analysis of the use of cement to anchor the femoral head prosthesis. *Journal of Bone and Joint Surgery (B)* **47**: 354–63.

Charnley J. (1966a) Using Teflon in arthroplasty of the hip joint. *Journal of Bone and Joint Surgery (A)* **48**: 819.

Charnley J. (1966b) The healing of human fractures in contact with self-curing acrylic cement. *Clinical Orthopaedics and Related Research* **47**: 157–63.

Charnley J. (1970) *Acrylic Cement in Orthopaedic Surgery.* Edinburgh: Livingstone.

Charnley J. (1972). *Post-Operative Infection after Total Hip Replacement with Special Reference to Air Contamination in the Operating Room.* Internal Publication No. 38. Wigan: Centre for Hip Surgery, Wrightington Hospital.

Charnley J. (1974) Total hip replacement. *Journal of the American Medical Association* **230**: 1025–8.

Charnley J. (1975a) [Several points on the technics for the prevention of the loosening of hip prosthesis] French. *Revue de Chirurgie Orthopédique et Réparatrice de l'Appareil Moteur* **61**(Suppl. 2): 73–6.

Charnley J. (1975b) The histology of loosening between acrylic cement and bone. *Journal of Bone and Joint Surgery (B)* **57**: 245.

Charnley J. (1979) *Low Friction Arthroplasty of the Hip: Theory and practice.* Berlin; New York, NY: Springer-Verlag.

Charnley J. (1983) The development of the centre for hip surgery at Wrightington hospital. In Swinburn W R. (ed.) *Wrightington Hospital, The story of the first 50 years.* Wrightington: Wrightington Hospital, 36–44.

Charnley J, Eftekhar N. (1969) Postoperative infection in total prosthetic replacement arthroplasty of the hip joint. With special reference to the bacterial content of the air of the operating room. *British Journal of Surgery* **56**: 641–9.

Charnley J, Ferreira A de S D. (1964) Transplantation of the greater trochanter in arthroplasty of the hip. *Journal of Bone and Joint Surgery (B)* **46**: 191–7.

Charnley J, Kamangar A, Longfield M D. (1969) The optimum size of prosthetic heads in relation to the wear of plastic sockets in total replacement of the hip. *Medical and Biological Engineering* **7**: 31–9.

Cholmeley J A. (1982) *A Brief History of the Royal National Orthopaedic Hospital from Its Origin in 1905 to 1982.* London: Royal National Orthopaedic Hospital.

Clarke I C. (1982) Symposium on surface replacement arthroplasty of the hip: Biomechanics: mutifactorial design choices – an essential compromise? *Orthopedic Clinics of North America* **13**: 681–707.

Cobb A G, Schmalzreid T P. (2006) The clinical significance of metal ion release from cobalt-chromium metal-on-metal hip joint arthroplasty. *Proceedings of the Institution of Mechanical Engineers. Part H, Journal of Engineering in Medicine* **220**: 385–98.

Coleman R F, Herrington J, Scales J T. (1973) Concentration of wear products in hair, blood and urine after total hip replacement. *British Medical Journal* **i**: 527–9.

Cooter R, Pickstone J V. (eds) (2002) *Companion to Medicine in the Twentieth Century.* Routledge World Reference Series. London: Routledge.

Costantino P D, Friedman C D, Jones K, Chow L C, Pelzer H J, Sisson G A. (1991) Hydroxyapatite cement, I: basic chemistry and histologic properties. *Archives of Otolaryngology, Head and Neck Surgery* **117**: 379–84.

Cotella L, Railton G T, Nunn D, Freeman M A R, Revell P A. (1990) ICLH double-cup arthroplasty, 1980–87. *Journal of Arthroplasty* **5**: 349–57.

Crout D H, Corkill J A, James M L, Ling R S M. (1979) Methylmethacrylate metabolism in man. The hydrolysis of methylmethacrylate to methacrylic acid during total hip replacement. *Clinical Orthopaedics and Related Research* **141**: 90–5.

Dandy D J, Theodorou B C. (1975) The management of local complications of total hip replacement by the McKee–Farrar technique. *Journal of Bone and Joint Surgery (B)* **57**: 30–5.

Daniel J, Ziaee H, Salama A, Pradhan C, McMinn D J. (2006) The effect of the diameter of metal-on-metal bearings on systemic exposure to cobalt and chromium. *Journal of Bone and Joint Surgery (B)* **88**: 443–8.

D'Arcy E J, Fell R H, Ansell B M, Arden G P. (1976) Ketamine and juvenile chronic polyarthritis (Still's disease). Anaesthetic problems in Still's disease and allied disorders. *Anaesthesia* **31**: 624–32.

Decoulx J. (1975) [Charnley–Müller prosthesis. Unusual problems of diagnosing loosening and techniques of resealing total prosthesis] French. *Revue de Chirurgie Orthopédique et Réparatrice de l'Appareil Moteur* **61**: 90–6.

Department of Health and Social Security (DHSS) and Medical Research Council (MRC), Joint Working Party. (1972). *Ventilation in Operating Suites: Report.* London: Medical Research Council.

Dobbs H S. (1980) Survivorship of total hip replacements. *Journal of Bone and Joint Surgery (B)* **62**: 168–73.

Dorr L D, Bechtol C O, Watkins R G, Wan Z. (2000) Radiographic anatomic structure of the arthritic acetabulum and its influence on total hip arthroplasty. *Journal of Arthroplasty* **15**: 890–900.

Dowson D. (ed.) (1998) *Advances in Medical Tribology: Orthopaedic implants and implant materials.* Bury St Edmunds: Mechanical Engineering Publications.

Dowson D. (2001) New joints for the Millennium: wear control in total replacement hip joints. *Proceedings of the Institution of Mechanical Engineers. Part H, Journal of Engineering in Medicine* **215**: 335–58.

Dowson D, Wright V. (1978) Bio-engineering at Leeds. *Engineering in Medicine, Institute of Mechanical Engineering* **7**: 63–5.

Dowson D, Wright V. (eds) (1981) *An Introduction to the Biomechanics of Joints and Joint Replacement.* London: Mechanical Engineering Publications.

Duff-Barclay I, Scales J T, Wilson J N. (1966) Biomechanics. The development of the Stanmore total hip replacement. *Proceedings of the Royal Society of Medicine* **59**: 948–51.

Elson R A, Jephcott A E, McGechie D B, Verettas D. (1977a) Antibiotic-loaded acrylic cement. *Journal of Bone and Joint Surgery (B)* **59**: 200–5.

Elson R A, Jephcott A E, McGechie D B, Verettas D. (1977b) Bacterial infection and acrylic cement in the rat. *Journal of Bone and Joint Surgery (B)* **59**: 452–7.

Elves M W, Wilson J N, Scales J T, Kemp H B. (1975) Incidence of metal sensitivity in patients with total joint replacements. *British Medical Journal* **iv**: 376–8.

Enright D. (ed.) (2001) *The Wicked Wit of Winston Churchill.* London: Michael O'Mara.

Erli H J, Marx R, Paar O, Niethard F U, Weber M, Wirtz D C. (2003) Surface pretreatments for medical application of adhesion. *Biomedical Engineering Online* **2**: 15.

Evans E M, Freeman M A R, Miller A J, Vernon-Roberts B. (1974) Metal sensitivity as a cause of bone necrosis and loosening of the prosthesis in total joint replacement. *Journal of Bone and Joint Surgery (B)* **56**: 626–42

Fang H-W, Hsu S M, Sengers J V. (2003) *Ultra-High Molecular Weight Polyethylene Wear Particle Effects on Bioactivity.* Department of Commerce, National Institute of Standards and Technology Special Publication 1002. Washington, DC: US Government Printing Office.

Faulkner A. (2002) Casing the joint: the material development of artificial hips, in Ott K, Serlin D, Mihm S. (eds) *Artificial Parts, Practical Lives: Modern histories of prosthetics.* New York, NY: New York University Press, 199–226.

Faulkner A, Kennedy L G, Baxter K, Donovan J, Wilkinson M, Bevan G. (1998) Effectiveness of hip prostheses in primary total hip replacement: a critical review of evidence and an economic model. *Health Technology Assessment* **2**(6): 1–134. For details of the series from the National Coordinating Centre for Health Technology Assessment, see www.hta.nhsweb.nhs.uk/projectdata/3_publication_listings_ALL.asp (visited 30 October 2006).

Fender D, Harper W M, Gregg P J. (2000) The Trent regional arthroplasty study. Experiences with a hip register. *Journal of Bone and Joint Surgery (B)* **82**: 944–7.

Fisher J, Hu X Q, Stewart T D, Williams S, Tipper J L, Ingham E, Stone M H, Davies C, Hatto P, Bolton J, Riley M, Hardaker C, Isaac G H, Berry G. (2004) Wear of surface engineered metal-on-metal hip prostheses. *Journal of Materials Science. Materials in Medicine* **15**: 225–35.

Fitzpatrick R, Lodge M, Shortall E, Dawson J, Sculpher M, Carr A, Murray D, Britton A, Morris R, Briggs A. (1998) Primary total hip replacement surgery: a systematic review of outcomes and modelling of cost-effectiveness associated with different prostheses. *Health Technology Assessment* **2**(20): 1–60. For details of the series from the National Coordinating Centre for Health Technology Assessment, see www.hta.nhsweb.nhs.uk/projectdata/3_publication_listings_ALL.asp (visited 30 October 2006).

Foreman-Peck J. (1995) *Smith & Nephew in the Health Care Industry.* Aldershot: Edward Elgar Publishing Ltd.

Fowler J L, Gie G A, Lee A J, Ling R S M. (1988) Experience with the Exeter total hip replacement since 1970. *Orthopedic Clinics of North America* **19**: 477–89. Erratum in: *Orthopedic Clinics of North America* (1989) **20**: preceding 519.

Freeman M A R. (ed.) (1973) *Adult Articular Cartilage.* London: Pitman. [2nd edn, Tunbridge Wells: Pitman Medical, 1979].

Freeman M A R. (ed.) (1978a) Total surface replacement hip arthroplasty. *Clinical Orthopaedics and Related Research* **134**: 2–371.

Freeman M A R. (1978b) Some anatomical and mechanical considerations relevant to the surface replacement of the femoral head. *Clinical Orthopaedics and Related Research* **134**: 19–24.

Freeman M A R, Bradley G W. (1982) ICLH double-cup arthroplasty. *Orthopedic Clinics of North America* **13**: 799–811.

Freeman M A R, Brown G C. (1978) ICLH cemented double-cup hip replacement. *Archives of Orthopaedic and Traumatic Surgery* **92**: 191–8.

Freeman M A R, Cameron H U, Brown G C. (1978) Cemented double-cup arthroplasty of the hip: a 5 year experience with the ICLH prosthesis. *Clinical Orthopaedics and Related Research* **134**: 45–52.

Freeman M A R, Rasmussen G L, Choy W S. (1985) Replacement of the acetabulum with pegged press-fit components. *Hip* (1985): 261–8.

Freeman M A R, Swanson S A V, Heath J C. (1969a) The production characterization and biological significance of the wear particles produced *in vitro* from cobalt-chromium-molybdenum total joint-replacement prostheses. *British Journal of Surgery* **56**: 701.

Freeman M A R, Swanson S A V, Heath J C. (1969b) Study of the wear particles produced from cobalt-chromium-molybdenum-manganese total joint replacement prostheses. *Annals of the Rheumatic Diseases* **28** (Suppl.): 29.

Freeman M A R, Swanson S A V, Day W H, Thomas R J. (1975) Proceedings: conservative total replacement of the hip. *Journal of Bone and Joint Surgery (B)* **57**: 114.

Geller J A, Malchau H, Bragdon C, Greene M, Harris W H, Freiberg A A. (2006) Large diameter femoral heads on highly cross-linked polyethylene: minimum 3-year results. *Clinical Orthopaedics and Related Research* **447**: 53–9.

Girdlestone G R. (1943) Acute pyogenic arthritis of the hip: an operation giving free access and effective drainage. *Lancet* **i**: 419–2. [A facsimile was published in *Clinical Orthopaedics and Related Research*, 1982, **170**: 3–7.]

Girdlestone G R, Somerville E W. (1952) *Tuberculosis of Bone and Joint*, 2nd edn. London: Oxford University Press. [3rd rev. edn, revised by E W Somerville and M C Wilkinson. London: Oxford University Press, 1965].

Glück T. (1891) Referat über die durch das moderne chirurgische Experiment gewormen positiven Resultate, betreffend die Naht und den Ersatz von Defekten hüherer Gewebe, sowie über die Verwertung resorbirbarer ünd lebendiger Tampons in der chirurgie. *Archiver klinische Chirurgie* **41**: 187–239.

Glyn-Jones S, Gill H S, McLardy-Smith P, Murray D W. (2004) A RSA study of the Birmingham reSurfacing Arthroplasty. International Society for Technology in Arthoplasty Oxford, England, 25–28 September 2002. *Journal of Bone and Joint Surgery (B)* **86**: 19.

Godsiff S, Emery R, Heywood-Waddington M, Thomas T. (1992) Cemented versus uncemented femoral components in the Ring hip prosthesis. *Journal of Bone and Joint Surgery (B)* **74**: 822–4.

Gomez P F, Morcuende J A. (2005a) Early attempts at hip arthroplasty – 1700s to 1950s. *Iowa Orthopaedic Journal* **25**: 25–9.

Gomez P F, Morcuende J A. (2005b) A historical and economic perspective on Sir John Charnley, Chas F Thackray Ltd, and the early arthroplasty industry. *Iowa Orthopaedic Journal* **25**: 30–7.

Grigoris P, Roberts P, McMinn D J, Villar R N. (1993) A technique for removing an intrapelvic acetabular cup. *Journal of Bone and Joint Surgery (B)* **75**: 25–7.

Haboush E J. (1953) A new operation for arthroplasty of the hip based on biomechanics, photoelasticity, fast-setting dental acrylic, and other considerations. *Bulletin of the Hospital for Joint Diseases* **14**: 242–77. [A facsimile was published in *Bulletin of the Hospital for Joint Diseases,* 1996, **55:** 95–111.]

Halliday B R, English H W, Timperley A J, Gie G A, Ling R S. (2003) Femoral impaction grafting with cement in revision total hip replacement. Evolution of the technique and results. *Journal of Bone and Joint Surgery (B)* **85**: 809–17.

Hampson P. (2004) John Tracey Scales. *British Medical Journal* **328**: 714.

Hardinge K. (1982) The direct lateral approach to the hip. *Journal of Bone and Joint Surgery (B)* **64**: 17–19.

Harper W M, Abrams K, Elson R. (1998) Correspondence: lessons of a hip failure. Register exists in Trent region. *British Medical Journal* **316**: 1985–6.

Hassan T, Birtwistle S, Power R A, Harper W M. (2000) Revision hip arthroplasty activity in a single UK health region: an audit of 1265 cases. *Annals of the Royal College of Surgeons of England* **82**: 283–6.

Heath J C, Freeman M A R, Swanson S A V. (1971) Carcinogenic properties of wear particles from prostheses made in cobalt-chromium alloy. *Lancet* **i**: 564–6.

Hernandez-Vaquero D. (1987) Mechanical failure in double-cup arthroplasty of the hip. *International Orthopaedics* **11**: 301–5.

Higuchi F, Gotoh M, Yamaguchi N, Suzuki R, Kunou Y, Ooishi K, Nagata K. (2003) Minimally invasive uncemented total hip arthroplasty through an anterolateral approach with a shorter skin incision. *Journal of Orthopaedic Science* **8**: 812–17.

Hill C, Flamant R, Mazas F, Everard J. (1981) Prophylactic cefazolin versus placebo in total hip replacement. Report of a multicentre double-blind randomized trial. *Lancet* **i**: 795–7.

Howie D W, McCalden R W, Nawana N S, Costi K, Pearcy M J, Subramanian C. (2005) The long-term wear of retrieved McKee–Farrar metal-on-metal total hip prostheses. *Journal of Arthroplasty* **20**: 350–7.

Howorth F H. (1985) Prevention of airborne infection during surgery. *Lancet* **i**: 386–8.

Howorth H. (2002) The evolution of ultra clean air systems for surgery, in Faux J C. (ed.) *After Charnley.* Preston: The John Charnley Trust and Colt Books Ltd, 125–37.

Hughes S P F. (1988) The role of antibiotics in preventing infections following total hip replacement. *Journal of Hospital Infection* **11**(Suppl. C): 41–7.

Hughes S P F, Sweetnam R. (eds) (1980) *The Basis and Practice of Orthopaedics.* London: Heinemann Medical.

Hungerford D S. (2005) The relationship between the American Association of Hip and Knee Surgeons and the *Journal of Arthroplasty. Journal of Arthroplasty* **20**: 6.

Inman V T. (1947) Functional aspects of the abductor muscles of the hip. *Journal of Bone and Joint Surgery (A)* **29**: 19.

Institution of Mechanical Engineers, Lubrication and Wear Group with the British Orthopaedic Association. (1967) Lubrication and wear in living and artificial human joints: a symposium, 7 April 1967. *Proceedings of the Institution of Mechanical Engineers, Part J, Journal of Engineering Tribology* **181**: part 3J.

Johnston R. (1981) The part luck played in the development of the plastic hip. [journal name not recorded on cutting] (3 December 1981): 24 [cutting provided by Mr Harry Craven].

Jolles B M, Bogoch E R. (2006) Posterior versus lateral surgical approach for total hip arthroplasty in adults with osteoarthritis. *Cochrane Database of Systematic Reviews* (3): CD003828. Freely available at www.mrw.interscience.wiley.com/cochrane/clsysrev/articles/CD003828/frame.html (visited 30 January 2007).

Jones J. (2000) National register will monitor hip replacements. *British Medical Journal* **320**: 1163.

Joosten U, Joist A, Gosheger G, Liljenqvist U, Brandt B, von Eiff C. (2005) Effectiveness of hydroxyapatite-vancomycin bone cement in the treatment of *Staphylococcus aureus*-induced chronic osteomyelitis. *Biomaterials* **26**: 5251–8.

Judet J. (1947) Prosthèses en résine acrylic. *Mémoires, Académie de Chirurgie* **73**: 561.

Judet J, Judet R. (1950) The use of an artificial femoral head for arthroplasty of the hip joint. *Journal of Bone and Joint Surgery* **32**-B: 166–73. Originally described in Judet (1947).

Kamerer D B, Hirsch B E, Snyderman C H, Costantino P, Friedman C D. (1994) Hydroxyapatite cement: a new method for achieving watertight closure in transtemporal surgery. *American Journal of Otology* **15**: 47–9.

Kenedi R M, Cowden J M, in association with J T Scales. (eds). (1976) *Bed Sore Biomechanics: Proceedings of a seminar on tissue viability and clinical applications.* Organized in association with the Department of Biomedical Engineering, the Institute of Orthopaedics (University of London), the Royal National Orthopaedic Hospital, Stanmore, London, and held at the University of Strathclyde, Glasgow, in August 1975. London: Macmillan.

Kent J, Faulkner A. (2002) Regulating human implant technologies in Europe – understanding the new era in medical device regulation. *Health, Risk and Society* **4**: 189–209.

Kiaer S, with Jansen K, Krogh-Poulsen W, Henrichsen E. (1953) Experimental investigation of the tissue reaction to acrylic plastics. Procès-verbaux, rapports, discussions et communications particulières: *Cinquième Congrès International de Chirurgie Orthopédique, Stockholm, 21–25 May 1951.* Bruxelles: Lielens, 534–6.

Klenerman L. (2002) Arthroplasty of the hip, in Klenerman L. (ed.). *The Evolution of Orthopaedic Surgery.* London: The Royal Society of Medicine Press, 13–23.

Langston H H. (1947) The Brittain method of arthrodesis of the hip. *Proceedings of the Royal Society of Medicine* **40**: 895–8.

Lalor P A, Revell P A, Gray A B, Wright S, Railton G T, Freeman M A R. (1991) Sensitivity to titanium. A cause of implant failure? *Journal of Bone and Joint Surgery (B)* **73**: 25–8.

Lawrence G. (ed.) (1994) *Technologies of Modern Medicine.* London: Science Museum.

Lettin A W F. (2004) Obituary: Professor John Scales. *The Times* (17 February): 61.

Levack B, Freeman M A R, de Alencar P G. (1986) Double cup replacement of the hip: development and current results up to 1984, in Sevastik J, Goldie I. (eds) *The Young Patient with Degenerative Hip Disease.* Stockholm: Almqvist & Wiksell, 175–80.

Li S, Burstein A H. (1994) Ultra-high molecular weight polyethylene. The material and its use in total joint implants. *Journal of Bone and Joint Surgery (A)* **76**: 1080–90.

Lidwell O M. (1990) The microbiology of air. In Linton A H, Dick H M. (eds) *Topley and Wilson's Principles of Bacteriology, Virology and Immunology. I. General Bacteriology and Immunity.* 8th edn. London: Edward Arnold, 226–41.

Lidwell O M. (1993) Sir John Charnley, surgeon (1911–82): the control of infection after total joint replacement. *Journal of Hospital Infection* **23**: 5–15.

Lidwell O M, Williams R E. (1960) The ventilation of operating theatres. *Journal of Hygiene* **58**: 449–64.

Lidwell O M, Lowbury E J L, Whyte W, Blowers R, Stanley S J, Lowe D. (1982) Effect of ultraclean air in operating rooms on deep sepsis in the joint after total hip or knee replacement: a randomized study. *British Medical Journal* **285**: 10–14.

Lidwell O M, Lowbury E J L, Whyte W, Blowers R, Stanley S J, Lowe D. (1983) Correspondence: ventilation in operating rooms. *British Medical Journal* **286**: 1214–15.

Lidwell O M, Elson R A, Lowbury E J L, Whyte W, Blowers R, Stanley S J, Lowe D. (1987) Ultraclean air and antibiotics for prevention of postoperative infection. A multicenter study of 8052 joint replacement operations. *Acta Orthopaedica Scandinavica* **58**: 4–13.

Lee A J, Ling R S M. (1974) A device to improve the extrusion of bone cement into the bone of the acetabulum in the replacement of the hip joint. *Biomedical Engineering* **9**: 522–4.

Lee A J, Ling R S M, Vangala S S. (1978) Some clinically relevant variables affecting the mechanical behaviour of bone cement. *Archives of Orthopaedic and Trauma Surgery* **92**: 1–18.

Ling R S M. (1997) *The History and Development of the Exeter Hip.* London: Howmedica.

Lowbury E J L, Lidwell O M. (1978) Multi-hospital trial on the use of ultraclean air systems in orthopaedic operating rooms to reduce infection: preliminary communication. *Journal of the Royal Society of Medicine* **71**: 800–6.

Löwy I. (ed.) (1993) *Medicine and Change: Historical and sociological studies of medical innovation.* Montrouge, France: John Libbey Eurotext.

Malchau H. (1996) *Swedish National Hip Register*. Göteborg: Department of Orthopaedics, University of Göteborg. For further details, see www.jru. orthop.gu.se/ (visited 7 June 2006).

Malchau H, Herberts P, Eisler T, Garellick G, Söderman P. (2002) The Swedish total hip replacement register. *Journal of Bone and Joint Surgery (A)* **84**: 2–20.

Markolf K L, Hirschowitz D L, Amstutz H C. (1979) Mechanical stability of the greater trochanter following osteotomy and reattachment by wiring. *Clinical Orthopaedics and Related Research* **141**: 111–21.

McCaskie A W, Richardson J B, Gregg P J. (1998) Further uses of polymethylmethacrylate in orthopaedic surgery. *Journal of the Royal College of Surgeons of Edinburgh* **43**: 37–9.

McKee G K. (1951) Open reduction and internal fixation in the treatment of fractures. *Medical Press* **225**: 577–81.

McKee G K. (1953) The use of wire rings for the fixation of spinal grafts. *Journal of Bone and Joint Surgery (B)* **35**: 258–9.

McKee G K. (1958) Two demonstrations given at a meeting of the RSM section on orthopaedics, 22 March 1958, at the Norfolk and Norwich Hospital, Norwich. 1. The use and development of an artificial hip joint (film); 2. Plastic disc supports. *Proceedings of the Royal Society of Medicine* **51**: 879–84.

McKee G K. (1966) Total hip replacement for advanced coxarthrosis. Extract from *Programme for the Société Internationale de Chirurgie Orthopédique et de Traumatologie* (SICOT) *Dixieme Congrès International de Chirurgie Orthopédique et de Traumatologie*, 4–9 September 1966. Paris: SICOT, 320–28.

McKee G K. (1967) Total prosthetic replacement of the hip. *Physiotherapy* **53**: 412–15.

McKee G K. (1974) The Norwich method of total hip replacement: development and main indications. *Annals of the Royal College of Surgeons of England* **54**: 53–62.

McKee G K. (1982) Total hip replacement – past, present and future. *Biomaterials* **3**: 130–5.

McKee G K, Chen S C. (1973) The statistics of the McKee–Farrar method of total hip replacement. *Clinical Orthopaedics* **95**: 26–33.

McKee G K, Watson-Farrar J. (1966) Replacement of arthritic hips by the McKee–Farrar prosthesis. *Journal of Bone and Joint Surgery (B)* **48**: 245–59.

McMinn D W. (2003) Development of metal/metal hip resurfacing [abstract]. *Hip* **13**: 41–3.

McMinn D J W, Daniel J. (2006) History and modern concepts in surface replacement. *Proceedings of the Institution of Mechanical Engineers, Part H, Journal of Engineering in Medicine* **220**: 239–51.

McMinn D J W, Daniel J, Ziaee H. (2005) Controversial topics in orthopaedics: metal-on-metal. *Annals of the Royal College of Surgeons of England* **87**: 411–15.

McMinn D J W, Roberts P, Forward G R. (1991) A new approach to the hip for revision surgery. *Journal of Bone and Joint Surgery (B)* **73**-B: 899–901.

McMinn D J W, Treacy R, Lin K, Pynsent P. (1996) Metal-on-metal surface replacement of the hip. Experience of the McMinn prosthesis. *Clinical Orthopaedics and Related Research* **329**: S89–S98.

Medical Research Council (MRC), Joint Working Party of the DHSS and MRC. (1972). *Ventilation in Operating Suites. Report of the Joint Working Party of the DHSS and MRC*. London: MRC.

Meers P D. (1983a) Editorial: ventilation in operating rooms. *British Medical Journal* **286**: 244–5.

Meers P D. (1983b) Correspondence: ventilation in operating rooms. *British Medical Journal* **286**: 1215.

Metcalfe J S, Pickstone J V. (2006) Replacing hips and lenses: surgery, industry and innovation in postwar Britain. In Webster A. (ed.) *New Technologies in Health Care: Challenge, change and innovation*. Basingstoke: Palgrave, 146–60.

Moore A T. (1952) Metal hip joint, a new self-locking Vitallium prosthesis. *Southern Medical Journal* **45**: 1015–19.

Moore A T. (1957) The self-locking metal hip prosthesis. *Journal of Bone and Joint Surgery (A)* **39**: 811–27.

Moore A T, Bohlman H R. (1943) Metal hip joint, a case report. *Journal of Bone and Joint Surgery (A)* **25**: 688–92.

Müller M E, Allgöwer M, Willenegger H. (1965) *Technique of Internal Fixation of Fractures.* Berlin: Springer-Verlag.

National Audit Office. (2000) *NHS Executive: Hip Replacements: Getting it right first time. A report by the Comptroller and Auditor General.* House of Commons papers, Session 1999–2000, HC 417. London: Stationery Office.

National Audit Office. (2003) *Hip Replacements: An update. A report by the Comptroller and Auditor General.* House of Commons papers, Session 2002–03, HC 956. London: Stationery Office.

NHS Centre for Reviews and Dissemination, University of York. (1996) Total hip replacement. *Effective Health Care* **2**: 1–12.

National Institute for Health and Clinical Excellence (NICE). (2000) *Guidance on the Selection of Prostheses for Primary Total Hip Replacement.* Technology Appraisal Guidance No. 2. London: NICE. Reviewed in April 2003, revised guidance at www.nice.org.uk/page.aspx?o=510 and TA44 on metal-on-metal hip resurfacing at www.nice.org.uk/page.aspx?o=33566 (both visited 1 August 2006).

Nicholson O R, Seddon H J. (1957) Nerve repair in civil practice; results of treatment of median and ulnar nerve lesions. *British Medical Journal* **ii**: 1065–71.

Oh I, Carlson C E, Tomford W W, Harris W H. (1978) Improved fixation of the femoral component after total hip replacement using a methacrylate intramedullary plug. *Journal of Bone and Joint Surgery (A)* **60**: 608–13.

Older J. (1986) A tribute to Sir John Charnley. *Clinical Orthopaedics* **211**: 23–9.

Older J. (2002) Charnley low-friction arthroplasty: a worldwide retrospective review at 15 to 20 years. *Journal of Arthroplasty* **17**: 675–80.

Olsson S S, Jernberger A, Tryggo D. (1981) Clinical and radiological long-term results after Charnley–Müller total hip replacement. A 5- to 10-year follow-up study with special reference to aseptic loosening. *Acta Orthopaedica Scandinavica* **52**: 531–42.

Owen R. (2006) James Noel Chalmers Barclay Wilson 1919–2006. *British Orthopaedic News* **33**: 54.

Pacheco V, Shelley P, Wroblewski B M. (1988) Mechanical loosening of the stem in Charnley arthroplasties. Identification of the 'at risk' factors. *Journal of Bone and Joint Surgery (B)* **70**: 596–9.

Padgett D E, Lipman J, Robie B, Nestor B J. (2006) Influence of total hip design on dislocation: a computer model and clinical analysis. *Clinical Orthopaedics and Related Research* **447**: 48–52.

Paltrinieri M, Trentani C. (1971) [Modification of hip arthroprosthesis] Italian. *La Chirurgia degli Organi di Movimento* **60**: 85–95.

Parker M, Gurusamy K. (2006) Arthroplasties (with and without bone cement) for proximal femoral fractures in adults. *Cochrane Database of Systematic Reviews* **3**: CD001706. Freely available at www.mrw.interscience.wiley.com/cochrane/clsysrev/articles/CD001706/frame.html (visited 30 January 2007).

Parsons D W. (1972) Total hip replacement, in Apley A G. (ed.) (1972) *Modern Trends in Orthopaedics 6*. London: Butterworths, PAGES.

Parsons D W, Seddon H J. (1968) The results of operations for disorders of the hip caused by poliomyelitis. *Journal of Bone and Joint Surgery (B)* **50**: 267–73.

Patterson F P, Brown C S. (1972) The McKee–Farrar total hip replacement. Preliminary results and complications of 368 operations performed in five general hospitals. *Journal of Bone and Joint Surgery (A)* **54**: 257–75.

Paul J P. (1966) Forces transmitted by joints in the human body. *Proceedings of the Institution of Mechanical Engineers. Part H, Journal of Engineering in Medicine* **181**: 8–15.

Paul J P. (1999) Strength requirements for internal and external prostheses. *Journal of Biomechanics* **32**: 381–93.

Paul J P. (2005) The history of musculoskeletal modelling in human gait. *Theoretical Issues in Ergonomics Science* **6**: 1–8.

Pauwels F. (1935) *Der Schenkelhalsbruch, ein mechanisches Problem.* Stuttgart: Enke.

Perka C, Fischer U, Taylor W R, Matziolis G. (2004) Developmental hip dysplasia treated with total hip arthroplasty with a straight stem and a threaded cup. *Journal of Bone and Joint Surgery (A)* **86**: 312–19.

Phillips H, Cole P V, Lettin A W F. (1971) Cardiovascular effects of implanted acrylic bone cement. *British Medical Journal* **iii**: 460–1.

Phillips H, Lettin A W F, Cole P V. (1973) Communication: cardiovascular effects of implanted acrylic cement. *Journal of Bone and Joint Surgery (B)* **55**: 210.

Pickstone J V. (ed.) (1992) *Medical Innovations in Historical Perspective.* Basingstoke: Palgrave Macmillan.

Pickstone J V. (2000) *Ways of Knowing: A new history of science, technology and medicine.* Manchester: Manchester University Press; Chicago, IL: Chicago University Press, 2001.

Pickstone J V. (2006) Bones in Lancashire: towards long-term contextual analysis of medical technology. In Timmermann C, Anderson J. (eds) *Devices and Designs: Medical technologies in historical perspective.* Houndmills: Palgrave Macmillan, 17–36.

Randall R L, Aoki S K, Olson P R, Bott S I. (2006) Complications of cemented long-stem hip arthroplasties in metastatic bone disease. *Clinical Orthopaedics and Related Research* **443**: 287–95.

Renner C. (1925) Die Shenton-Linie. *Zentralblatt für Chirurgie* **52**: 2875–6.

Ring P A. (1968) Complete replacement arthroplasty of the hip by the Ring prosthesis. *Journal of Bone and Joint Surgery (B)* **50**: 720–31.

Ring P A. (1970a) Correspondence: Super-specialization in surgery. *British Medical Journal* **iii**: 45.

Ring P A. (1970b) Total replacement of the hip. *Clinical Orthopaedics and Related Research* **72**: 161–8.

Ring P A. (1974) Total replacement of the hip joint. A review of a thousand operations. *Journal of Bone and Joint Surgery (B)* **56**: 44–58.

Ring P A. (1978) Five to fourteen year interim results of uncemented total hip arthroplasty. *Clinical Orthopaedics and Related Research* **137**: 87–95.

Ring P A. (1981) Uncemented total hip replacement. *Journal of the Royal Society of Medicine* **74**: 719–24.

Ring P A. (1983) Ring UPM total hip arthroplasty. *Clinical Orthopaedics and Related Research* **176**: 115–23.

Roberts P, Walters A J, McMinn D J. (1992) Diagnosing infection in hip replacements. The use of fine-needle aspiration and radiometric culture. *Journal of Bone and Joint Surgery (B)* **74**: 265–9.

Roberts P, Chan D, Grimer R J, Sneath R S, Scales J T. (1991) Prosthetic replacement of the distal femur for primary bone tumours. *Journal of Bone and Joint Surgery (B)* **73**: 762–9.

Salvati E A, Robinson R P, Zeno S M, Koslin B L, Brause B D, Wilson P D Jr. (1982) Infection rates after 3175 total hip and total knee replacements performed with and without a horizontal unidirectional filtered air-flow system. *Journal of Bone and Joint Surgery (A)* **64**: 525–35.

Scales J T. (1965) The development of British Standards for surgical implants. *Journal of Bone and Joint Surgery (B)* 47: 111–17.

Scales J T. (1966–7) Arthroplasty of the hip using foreign materials: a history. *Proceedings of the Institution of Mechanical Engineers Part H, Journal of Engineering in Medicine* **181**: 63–84.

Scales J T. (1983) Editorial: prosthetic replacement of the femoral head for femoral neck fractures: which design? *Journal of Bone and Joint Surgery (B)* **65**: 530–2.

Scales J T, Wilson J N. (1969) Some aspects of the development of the Stanmore total hip joint prosthesis. *Reconstruction Surgery and Traumatology* **11**: 20–39.

Scales J T, Duff-Barclay I, Burrows J H. (1965) Some engineering and medical problems associated with massive bone replacement. In Kenedi R M. (ed.) *Biomechanics and Related Bio-Engineering Topics.* Oxford: Pergamon Press, 205–39.

Schmalzried T P, Fowble V A, Ure K J, Amstutz H C. (1996) Metal-on-metal surface replacement of the hip. Technique, fixation and early results. *Clinical Orthopaedics and Related Research* **329** (Suppl.): S106–14.

Scottish Society for Contamination Control (S2C2). (2004a) Laminar flow in hospitals. 3a: Hospitals: Sir John Charnley. *S2C2 Cleanroom Monitor* **50**: 4–7. Freely available at www.s2c2.co.uk/monitor/tcm50.pdf (visited 18 October 2006).

S2C2. (2004b) Laminar flow in hospitals. 3b: Laminar Flow ORs. *S2C2 Cleanroom Monitor* **51**: 4–7. Freely available at www.s2c2.co.uk/monitor/tcm51.pdf (visited 18 October 2006).

Seddon H J. (1950) Peripheral nerve injuries in Great Britain during World War II: a review. *Archives of Neurology and Psychiatry* **63**: 171–3.

Seddon H J. (1967) In memoriam: Philip Wiles. *Journal of Bone and Joint Surgery (B)* **49**: 580–1.

Seddon H J, Scales J T. (1949) A polythene substitute for the upper two-thirds of the shaft of the femur. *Lancet* **ii**: 795.

Semlitsch M, Willert H G. (1997) Clinical wear behaviour of ultra-high molecular weight polyethylene cups paired with metal and ceramic ball heads in comparison to metal-on-metal pairings of hip joint replacements. *Proceedings of the Institution of Mechanical Engineers. Part H, Journal of Engineering in Medicine* **211**: 73–88.

Semlitsch M, Lehmann M, Weber H, Doerre E, Willert H G. (1977) New prospects for a prolonged functional life-span of artificial hip joints by using the material combination polyethylene/aluminium oxide ceramin/metal. *Journal of Biomedical Materials Research* **11**: 537–52.

Shen C, Dumbleton J H. (1974) The friction and wear behaviour of irradiated very high molecular weight polyethylene. *Wear* **30**: 349–64.

Smith-Petersen M N. (1939) Arthroplasty of the hip: a new method. *Journal of Bone and Joint Surgery* **21**: 269–88.

Somerville E W. (1982) *Displacement of the Hip in Childhood: Aetiology, management, and sequelae.* Berlin; New York, NY: Springer-Verlag.

Stansfield B W, Nicol A C, Paul J P, Kelly I G, Graichen F, Bergmann G. (2003) Direct comparison of calculated hip joint contact forces with those measured using instrumented implants. An evaluation of a three-dimensional mathematical model of the lower limb. *Journal of Biomechanics* **36**: 929–36.

Stanton J. (ed.) (2002) *Innovations in Health and Medicine: Diffusion and resistance in the Twentieth Century*, Routledge Studies in the Social History of Medicine. London and New York, NY: Routledge.

Stephenson P K, Freeman M A R, Revell P A, Germain J, Tuke M, Pirie C J. (1991) The effect of hydroxyapatite coating on ingrowth of bone into cavities in an implant. *Journal of Arthroplasty* **6**: 51–8.

Swanson R L, Evarts C M. (1984) Dual-lock total hip arthroplasty. A preliminary experience. *Clinical Orthopaedics and Related Research* **191**: 224–31.

Swanson S A V, Freeman M A R. (1977) *The Scientific Basis of Total Joint Replacement.* London: Pitman Medical.

Swanson S A V, Freeman M A R, Heath J C. (1973) Laboratory tests on total joint replacement prostheses. *Journal of Bone and Joint Surgery (B)* **55**: 759–73.

Sweetnam D R. (1981) A surveillance scheme with 'Recommended List' of artificial joints. *Health Trends* **13**: 43–4.

Taggart T, Kerry R M, Norman P, Stockley I. (2002) The use of vancomycin-impregnated cement beads in the management of infection of prosthetic joints. *Journal of Bone and Joint Surgery (B)* **84**: 70–2.

Tennent T D, Eastwood D M. (1998) Survival of the Judet hip prosthesis. *Journal of the Royal Society of Medicine* **91**: 385–6.

Thompson F R. (1952) Vitallium intramedullary hip prosthesis, preliminary report. *New York State Journal of Medicine* **52**: 3011–20.

Thompson F R. (1966) An essay on the development of arthroplasty of the hip. *Clinical Orthopaedics and Related Research* **44**: 73–82.

Timmermann C, Anderson J. (eds) (2006) *Devices and Designs: Medical technologies in historical perspective.* Houndmills: Palgrave Macmillan.

Trentani C, Olmi R. (1974) [Therapeutic trends in aseptic necrosis of the femoral head in adults] Italian. *La Chirurgia degli Organi di Movimento* **61**: 491–501.

Trentani C, Vaccarino F. (1978) The Paltrinieri–Trentani hip joint resurface arthroplasty. *Clinical Orthopaedics and Related Research* **134**: 36–40.

Venable C S, Stuck W G. (1943) Clinical uses of Vitallium. *Annals of Surgery* **117**: 772–82.

Wahlig H, Buchholz H W. (1972) [Experimental and clinical studies on the release of gentamicin from bone cement] German. *Der Chirurg; Zeitschrift für alle Gebiete der operativen Medizen* **43**: 441–5.

Wahlig H, Dingeldein E, Buchholz H W, Buchholz M, Bachmann F. (1984) Pharmacokinetic study of gentamicin-loaded cement in total hip replacements. Comparative effects of varying dosage. *Journal of Bone and Joint Surgery (B)* **66**: 175–9.

Wainwright P. (1997) *Opposite the Infirmary: A history of the Thackray company 1902–90.* Leeds: Medical Museum.

Walker P S. (1977) *Human Joints and Their Artificial Replacements.* Springfield, IL: Charles C Thomas Publisher.

Watson-Jones R. (1935) Fractures of the neck of the femur. *British Journal of Surgery* **23**: 787–808.

Watson-Jones Sir Reginald. (1976, 1982) *Fractures and Joint Injuries*, vol. 2. Fifth and sixth edn edited by Wilson J N. Edinburgh; New York, NY: Churchill Livingstone.

Waugh W. (1990) *John Charnley: The man and the hip.* London: Springer-Verlag, 1990.

Webster A. (ed.) (2006) *New Technologies in Health Care: Challenge, change and innovation.* Basingstoke: Palgrave.

Weightman B, Swanson S A V, Isaac G H, Wroblewski B M. (1991) Polyethylene wear from retrieved acetabular cups. *Journal of Bone and Joint Surgery (B)* **73**: 806–10.

Weinrauch P C L, Moore W R, Shooter D R, Wilkinson M P R, Bonrath E M, Dedy N J, McMeniman T J, Jabur M K A, Whitehouse S L, Crawford R W. (2006) Early prosthetic complications after unipolar hemiarthroplasty. *ANZ Journal of Surgery* **76**: 432–5.

Wheble V H. (1994) Design validation through clinical testing, in van Gruting C W D. (ed.) *Medical Devices: International perspectives on health and safety.* Amsterdam: Elsevier, 54–74.

Whyte W. (2001) *Cleanroom Technology: Fundamentals of design, testing and operation.* New York, NY: John Wiley & Sons.

Wiles P. (1958) The surgery of the osteo-arthritic hip. *British Journal of Surgery* **45**: 488–97.

Wiles P, Sweetnam R. (1965) *Essentials of Orthopaedics*, 4th edn. London: Churchill.

Willert H G. (1977) Reactions of the articular capsule to wear products of artificial joint prostheses. *Journal of Biomedical Materials Research* **11**: 157–64.

Willert H G, Semlitsch M. (1976) Tissue reactions to plastic and metallic wear products of joint endoprostheses. In Gschwend N, Debrunner H U. (eds) *Total Hip Prosthesis*. Bern: H Huber, 205–39.

Willert H G, Ludwig J, Semlitsch M. (1974) Reaction of bone to methacrylate after hip arthroplasty: a long-term gross, light microscopic, and scanning electron microscopic study. *Journal of Bone and Joint Surgery (A)* **56**: 1368–82.

Wilson J N. (1953) Sarcoma of the upper end of the fibula simulating osteomyelitis. *British Journal of Surgery* **40**: 399–400.

Wilson J N. (1971) Prosthetic replacement of long bone for tumour (two cases). *Proceedings of the Royal Society of Medicine* **64**: 716–17.

Wilson J N, Scales J T. (1973) The Stanmore metal-on-metal total hip prosthesis using a three pin type cup. A follow-up of 100 arthroplasties over nine years. *Clinical Orthopaedics and Related Research* **95**: 239–49.

Wilson P D Jr, Amstutz H C, Czerniecki A, Salvati E A, Mendes D G. (1972) Total hip replacement with fixation by acrylic cement. A preliminary study of 100 consecutive McKee-Farrar prosthetic replacements. *Journal of Bone and Joint Surgery (A)* **54**: 207–36.

Wroblewski B M. (1986) Charnley low-friction arthroplasty. Review of the past, present status, and prospects for the future. *Clinical Orthopaedics and Related Research* **210**: 37–42.

Wroblewski B M. (1990) *Revision Surgery in Total Hip Arthroplasty*. London; New York, NY: Springer-Verlag.

Wroblewski B M. (1997) Wear of the high-density polyethylene socket in total hip arthroplasty and its role in endosteal cavitation. *Proceedings of the Institution of Mechanical Engineers. Part H, Journal of Engineering in Medicine* **211**: 109–18.

Wroblewski B M. (2002) Professor Sir John Charnley (1911–82). *Rheumatology* **41**: 824–5.

Wroblewski B M, Siney P D, Fleming P A. (2002) Charnley low-frictional torque arthroplasty in patients under the age of 51 years. Follow-up to 33 years. *Journal of Bone and Joint Surgery (B)* **84**: 540–3.

Wroblewski B M, Siney P D, Fleming P A. (2004) Wear of the cup in the Charnley LFA in the young patient. *Journal of Bone and Joint Surgery (B)* **86**: 498–503.

Wroblewski B M, Raut V V, Siney P D, Evans A R. (1995) An intrapelvic polytetrafluoroethylene granuloma. *Orthopaedics* (International edn) **3**: 439–44.

Biographical notes*

Sir Christopher Booth
Kt FRCP (b. 1924) trained as a gastroenterologist and was Professor of Medicine at the Royal Postgraduate Medical School, Hammersmith Hospital, London, from 1966 to 1977 and Director of the Medical Research Council's Clinical Research Centre, Northwick Park Hospital, Harrow, from 1978 to 1988. He was the first Convenor of the Wellcome Trust's History of Twentieth Century Medicine Group, from 1990 to 1996, and Harveian Librarian at the Royal College of Physicians from 1989 to 1997.

Mr Harold Jackson Burrows
CBE FRCS LRCP (1902–81), son of Harold Burrows FRCS, trained at St Bartholomew's Hospital, London, where he had house duties, returning to Cambridge on a Beaverbrook Research Scholarship from the Royal College of Surgeons to study tissue culture and later at the Rockefeller Institute, New York, NY. He was appointed surgical registrar at the RNOH in 1931, and chief assistant in the orthopaedic department at Bart's from 1931–36, and assistant orthopaedic surgeon from 1937 to 1948. He was Surgeon-Commander in the Royal Navy Volunteer Reserve during the war and was an active civilian consultant surgeon to the Royal Navy from 1949–77. He returned to Bart's as orthopaedic surgeon from 1948–67 and was a lecturer in orthopaedics there. He was Dean of the Institute of Orthopaedics, at the British Postgraduate Medical Federation, University of London, from 1946–64 and 1967–70; honorary orthopaedic surgeon to the National Hospital for Diseases of the Nervous System; and a consultant adviser to the Ministry of Health and Chairman of their Standing Advisory Committee on Artificial Limbs. He was President of the Orthopaedic Section of the Royal Society of Medicine; President of the BOA in 1966–67; and assistant editor, then deputy editor of the *Journal of Bone and Joint Surgery* until 1973. See Anonymous (1988).

* Contributors are asked to supply details; other entries are compiled from conventional biographical sources.

Lady (Jill) Charnley
Wife of Sir John Charnley.

Professor Sir John Charnley
Kt CBE DSc FRCS FRS
(1911–82), orthopaedic surgeon,
invented the low-friction hip
replacement in the early 1960s.
He served in the Royal Army
Medical Corps at Dunkirk and
in Cairo and was appointed
assistant orthopaedic surgeon,
Manchester Royal Infirmary, later
Consultant Orthopaedic Surgeon
at Wrightington Hospital, near
Wigan, Lancashire, from 1947 to
1980. He established and became
the first director of the Centre
for Hip Surgery, Wrightington
Hospital, in 1961. He was
Professor of Orthopaedic Surgery at
the University of Manchester from
1972 to 1976, later Emeritus. His
many honours and awards include
the honorary fellowship of BOA,
1981, and the Lister Medal of the
Royal College of Surgeons, 1975.
Following his death in 1982, Lady
Charnley established the John
Charnley Trust, which supports the
John Charnley Research Institute.
See Charnley (1950, 1960, 1983).
See also Wroblewski (2002) and
Figure 9.

Mr Tristram Charnley
Son of Sir John Charnley.

Professor Christopher Colton
MB FRCS FRCSEd (b. 1937)
trained at St Thomas' Hospital,
University of London. He was
Consultant in Orthopaedic and
Accident Surgery, Nottingham
University Hospital from
1973–97, and Special Professor in
Orthopaedic and Accident Surgery,
Faculty of Medicine, University
of Nottingham, from 1993 until
his retirement from the NHS in
1997, later Emeritus. He has been a
member of the BOA since 1970, its
President in 1995/6; and a member
of the Editorial Board of the
Journal of Bone and Joint Surgery in
1989–91 and 1994/5. He is now
an independent specialist in clinical
and medico–legal practice.

Mr Harry Craven
(1928–2007) started his
apprenticeship in engineering at
Walker Brothers (Wigan) Ltd,
engineers and mining machinery
manufacturers, in 1942, where
he worked until 1954. He joined
the Metal Box Company Ltd as a
management trainee until 1958,
when he became Chief Research
Technician for Mr John Charnley at
Wrightington Hospital, near Wigan.
There he designed and built many
components used by orthopaedic
surgeons. He moved to Liverpool
University in 1966 to set up the Bio-
Engineering Department testing the
loading of bone fractures, checked

by X-rays. In 1976 he went to the Groote Schuur Hospital, Cape Town, South Africa, returning to the UK to become works manager at Surgical Implant Engineering (SIE) in 1982, until it closed the following year. He started his own business making joints for 14 hospitals until he retired in 1995 due to ill health. See Figure 10.

Ms Clare Darrah

RGN DipSci (b. 1958) trained as a nurse at St Bartholomew's Hospital, London, from 1977–80, and has been Clinical Research Manager at the Institute of Orthopaedics, Norfolk and Norwich University Hospital, Norwich, since 1996. She conducts the joint review programme to provide long-term surveillance of hip and knee replacements. She is a founder member of the Arthroplasty Care Practitioners Association.

Mr Graham Deane

MB MSc FRCS (b. 1939) orthopaedic surgeon, graduated in biomechanics in 1970, was appointed Lecturer in Orthopaedics to the University of Oxford in 1971 and Consultant to the Oxford Orthopaedic Engineering Centre in 1973 at the Nuffield Orthopaedic Centre. He moved to Heatherwood and Wexham Park Hospitals [formerly the Windsor Group of Hospitals], in 1978 until

his retirement in 2002. His major interests and publications have been in biomechanics, orthotics and total joint replacements, particularly the knee. He has designed surgical devices, including two knee joint prostheses. He was Vice-Chairman of the Court of Examiners and Senior Examiner at the Royal College of Surgeons of England in 2000.

Professor Duncan Dowson

CBE PhD DSc FEng FRS (b. 1928) was Research Engineer at Sir W G Armstrong Whitworth Aircraft Co., from 1953 to 1954, then Lecturer in Mechanical Engineering in 1954, later Senior Lecturer, Reader and Professor of Engineering Fluid Mechanics and Tribology at the University of Leeds from 1966 until his retirement in 1993. He served as Head of Department of Mechanical Engineering (1987–92), Dean for International Relations (1987–93) and Pro-Vice Chancellor (1983–85). He was President of the Institution of Mechanical Engineers (1992–93), a Foreign Member Royal Swedish Academy and co-founder with Professor Verna Wright of the Leeds Bio-Engineering Group for the Study of Human Joints in 1966 and the Centre for Studies in Medical Engineering in 1971. See Dowson and Wright (1978, 1981).

Mrs Sheila Edwards
(b. 1947, née Wilson), 'Ginger' Wilson's daughter.

Mr Reg Elson
FRCS (b. 1930) qualified at Cambridge in 1954, having done clinical work at the London Hospital. Subsequently he trained as an orthopaedic trauma surgeon and was appointed to the Northern General Hospital in Sheffield in 1967 in charge of the trauma service there. As a result of a delay in rebuilding in Sheffield, he reverted to joint replacement surgery and in 1977 worked at the EndoKlinik in Hamburg, almost staying there permanently. He returned to Sheffield where a unit was established dealing with revision surgery, especially infected cases. He has been President of the European Hip Society and of the British Hip Society, and was a founder of the Cavendish Hip Fellowship Trust.

Dr Alex Faulkner
MA PhD (b. 1952), medical and healthcare sociologist, researches and writes about new medical technologies in the context of healthcare systems and health policy. He was appointed to the Department of Social Medicine at the University of Bristol from 1990 to 1999 and has been at Cardiff University's School of Social Sciences since 1999. He led a 'systematic review' of the performance of total hip replacements in 1998 See Faulkner *et al.* (1998); Faulkner (2002); Kent and Faulkner (2002).

Professor Michael Freeman
FRCS (b. 1931) trained at the London Hospital. Along with Alan Swanson, he was co-founder of the Biomechanics Unit, Imperial College, London, in 1964, appointed Consultant Orthopaedic Surgeon at the London Hospital from 1968 until his retirement in 1996 and Research Fellow at Imperial College, London from 1968 until 1979. He has been Honorary Consultant, Royal Hospitals NHS Trust, since 1996. He originated new surgical procedures for reconstruction and replacement arthritic hip, knee, ankle and foot joints. He was President of the International Hip Society from 1982 to 1985; the British Hip Society from 1989 to 1991; and the BOA from 1992 to 1993. See Freeman (ed.) (1973); Swanson and Freeman (eds) (1977).

Mrs Phyllis Hampson
(b. 1927) started work at the London Splint Company in 1944, moving in 1947 to work for Zimmer Orthopaedic Ltd (ZOL), Bridgend, South Wales, as non-

executive director. She returned to London in 1949 to start ZOL's sales office, was promoted to Sales Manager in 1958, Director of Sales in 1966 and Managing Director in 1968. ZOL was sold to Biomet in 1984 on the death of the owner, and Mrs Hampson retired in 1985.

Mr Kevin Hardinge

FRCS (b. 1939) qualified at Liverpool and held house and registrar posts at the Liverpool Royal Infirmary. He was appointed Consultant Orthopedic Surgeon at the Manchester Royal Infirmary, 1973–76; and has been Consultant Orthopedic Surgeon at the Wrightington Hospital, Wigan, since 1976; Honorary Lecturer in Orthopedics at the University of Manchester, since 1979; and Hunterian Professor at the Royal Society of Surgeons of England, since 1972.

Mr Mike Heywood-Waddington

MA FRCS (b. 1929) qualified at Cambridge; trained at Exeter, Stanmore and Great Ormond Street Hospital, London; and served with the Royal Air Force. He was Consultant in Orthopaedic and Traumatic Surgery to Mid-Essex and North Essex Health Authorities from 1967 to 1992 and Honorary Orthopaedic Consultant since 1992. He is a Founder Member of the British Hip Society and the British Orthopaedic Sports Trauma Association; a past President of the Orthopaedic Section of the Royal Society of Medicine; a Senior Fellow of the BOA and is Orthopaedic Surgeon to Essex County Cricket Club.

Mr Geoff King

(b. 1947) had multiple fractures following an accident involving a lorry in 1963, the treatment of which resulted in his interest in the health service. He worked in the NHS for 36 years, initially as a technician in the orthopaedic theatres in the Norfolk and Norwich Hospitals where the McKee and the McKee–Farrar hip joint replacements were developed. Latterly he was a general manager in the NHS before retiring in 2004 and had a hip replacement (the Birmingham re-surfacing double cup type, suitable for use in the 'younger' patient) in 2005.

Mr John Kirkup

FRCS DHMSA (b. 1928), orthopaedic surgeon and surgical historian, qualified at St Mary's Hospital, London, in 1952 and, after service in the Royal Navy, worked with Kenneth McKee at the Norfolk and Norwich Hospital from 1956 to 1958; John Charnley in 1959 and at the Bath and Wessex Orthopaedic Hospital from 1961 to 1964, becoming

Consultant Orthopaedic Surgeon to the Bath Clinical Area from 1964 until 1988. He introduced an ankle joint replacement in 1976. He was a UK Travelling Scholar (1964) and Honorary Archivist to the BOA (1980–2005); President of the British Orthopaedic Foot Surgical Society (1984); Brattstrom Lecturer to the Swedish Society for Rheumatoid Surgery (1985); and Vicary Lecturer (1976), Sir Arthur Keith Medallist (1998) at the Royal College of Surgeons of England and Honorary Curator of the Historical Instrument Collection there since 1980.

Mr K M N (Ravi) Kunzru

MS FRCS DHMSA (b. 1937) was Consultant Orthopaedic Surgeon at Whipps Cross University Hospital, London, from 1973 until his retirement in 1998, later Emeritus Consultant and Medical Historian. The final part of his training as Senior Registrar included working with Arden, Ansell, Maudsley and Swann on joint replacement, including children's joints, at the Windsor Group of Hospitals. He is current President of the History of Medicine Section of the Royal Society of Medicine (2005/06) and Vice President of the Medical Society of London (2005–7), Past President of the Hunterian Society (currently co-Curator of its collection); and Past President of the British Orthopaedic Foot and Ankle Surgery Society.

Mr W Alexander (Scottie) Law

OBE MD LRCP FRCS (1910–89) qualified at the London Hospital in 1935 with junior appointments in orthopaedic surgery there followed by war service in the RAMC, receiving the OBE for his military service. He returned to the London Hospital as consultant orthopaedic surgeon in 1947, later consultant to the Royal Masonic Hospital and the Italian Hospital, London, and associate surgeon to the Robert Jones and Agnes Hunt Hospital, Oswestry. He spent the year of 1948 with Smith-Petersen at the Massachusetts General Hospital, Boston, learning about cup arthroplasty, which he introduced on his return to London in 1949. He was President of the Orthopaedic Section of the Royal Society of Medicine.

Miss Betty Lee

RGN (b. 1925), trained in nursing at Mile End Hospital, London, in 1943, became a staff nurse in the male orthopaedic ward, Norfolk and Norwich Hospital, Norwich, from 1950 to 1953, a ward sister from 1953 to 1967, and was appointed to the teaching staff of the Broadland School of Nursing, Norwich, from 1967 until her retirement in 1985, including work on the RCN teaching course. She was Mr McKee's staff nurse and ward sister from 1950 until 1966.

Mr Alan Lettin

MS FRCS (b. 1931) qualified at University College Hospital, London, received his orthopaedic training at the RNOH and became lecturer and first assistant to Sir Hubert Seddon at the Institute of Orthopaedics. He was Consultant Orthopaedic Surgeon at St Bartholomew's Hospital, London, from 1967 to 1996 and the Royal National Orthopaedic Hospital, Stanmore, from 1968 to 1995. He collaborated with John Scales at the Institute of Orthopaedics, University of London, in the development and introduction of the Stanmore range of artificial joints and was responsible for the first total shoulder replacement in the world in 1970. He was President of the BOA (1994–95) and Vice-President of the Royal College of Surgeons (1995–97).

Professor Robin Ling

OBE HonFRCSEd FRCS (b. 1927), co-originator of the Exeter Hip, was educated in British Columbia, Oxford University and St Mary's Hospital, London. He was appointed Consultant Honorary Lecturer in the Department of Orthopaedic Surgery of the University of Edinburgh, 1960 to 1963; Consultant Orthopaedic Surgeon at the Royal Infirmary of Edinburgh and the Princess Margaret Rose Orthopaedic Hospital, Edinburgh, 1961 to 1963, and moved to the Princess Elizabeth Orthopaedic Centre, Exeter, Devon as Consultant Orthopaedic Surgeon in 1963 until 1991, which culminated in the implantation of the first Exeter Hip in the autumn of 1970. He set up a system to allow the prospective gathering of all data on hip arthroplasties from that time. He has been President of the British Orthopaedic Research Society, the BOA, the British Hip Society and the International Hip Society.

Mr Ken McKee

CBE FRCS (1905–1991), the first to replace a hip joint in 1951 by a reproducible method that others could use, qualified at St Bartholomew's Hospital, London, and trained in orthopaedic surgery at Chailey Heritage Hospital, Lewes, East Sussex, under Reginald Cheyne Elmslie (1878–1940), Sydney Limbrey Higgs (1892–1977) and Sam Brockman (1894–1977). He was Orthopaedic Registrar at Norfolk and Norwich Hospital from 1935 to 1939 and Consultant Orthopaedic Surgeon there from 1939 to 1971.

Dr Austin T Moore

MD (1899–1963), US orthopaedic surgeon, performed and reported the first metallic hip hemi-arthroplasty surgery in 1942. His original head and stem was made of the metal vitallium, about 12 inches long and was bolted to the cut end of the femoral shaft; a later version, the Austin Moore, is still used today for fractures of the femoral neck. See Moore and Bohlman (1943).

Dr Francis Neary

PhD (b. 1971) is a research associate in the Centre for the History of Science, Technology and Medicine at the University of Manchester. His recent research has been concerned with the history of twentieth-century medical technologies and he has curated exhibitions on joint replacement at the Royal College of Surgeons of England and at Wrightington Hospital, near Wigan in 2006.

Mr John Older

FRCSEd FRCS (b. 1935) qualified at Guy's Hospital, London and did his orthopaedic training in Bristol. He was a Senior Clinical Research Fellow, Toronto, Canada, before being appointed Consultant Orthopaedic Surgeon at the Royal Surrey County Hospital, Guildford, Surrey, from 1975 to 2001. He was a pupil, assistant and colleague of Sir John Charnley from 1978 to 1982 at the King Edward VII Hospital, Midhurst, West Sussex, where he remained until 2006, following the closure of the hospital. He has been Clinical Anatomist at King's College London Medical School, Guy's Campus, London, since 2001. He continues a special interest in primary and revision hip replacement surgery and continues to review the long-term results of the LFA. See Older (2002).

Professor John Paul

(b. 1927) was appointed in 1949 to the Department of Mechanical Engineering of the institution that was to become the University of Strathclyde, Glasgow. He became Senior Lecturer in Bioengineering in 1969, received a personal chair in 1972, and became Professor and Head of the Bioengineering Unit in 1978; Emeritus on his retirement in 1992, a position which he still holds. He has been Chairman of the International Standards Organization Sub-committee on Bone and Joint Replacements since 1992.

Professor John Pickstone

PhD (b. 1944) trained in biomedical sciences and in history and philosophy of science. Since 1974 he has worked in Manchester where he founded the Wellcome

Unit and the Centre for the History of Science, Technology and Medicine at the University of Manchester. Since 2002 he has been the Wellcome Research Professor at the Centre. His present projects include recent histories of cancer, the artificial hip and the NHS in Manchester. He also writes on the historical sociology of the history of science, technology and medicine. See Pickstone (2000); Cooter and Pickstone (eds) (2002).

Mr John Read

FRCSEd qualified at University College Hospital, London, and spent three years in the Royal Army Medical Corps as a Clinical Officer in surgery at the British Military Hospital and 33 General Hospitals in Hong Kong. He was appointed Registrar at the Sunderland Orthopaedic and Accident Hospital, later registrar to John Charnley at his new Centre for Hip Surgery at Wrightington Hospital; and senior registrar at the London Hospital. He was Consultant Orthopaedic Surgeon to the Harlow, Hertford and Harlow Hospitals, later Welwyn Garden City Hospital, continuing his special interest in primary and revision hip joint replacement surgery.

Mr Peter Ring

MS FRCS (b. 1922) was Consulting Orthopaedic Surgeon to the Redhill (Surrey) group of hospitals and Surgeon-in-Charge of the Joint Replacement Unit, Dorking Hospital, from 1959 to 1988.

Professor John Tracey Scales

OBE (1920–2004), designer of the Stanmore hip, was lecturer then reader at the Institute of Orthopaedics, Royal National Orthopaedic Hospital (RNOH), London and Stanmore, from 1952 to 1974. During this time he developed airstrip dressings. He was appointed Professor of Biomechanical Engineering in the University of London, in 1974, until his retirement in 1987, later Emeritus. He started the biomedical engineering department at the RNOH, the Institute of Orthopaedics, part of the University of London. He designed the Stanmore range of total joints for hips (with the assistance of Alan Lettin), knees, shoulders and elbows. He was honorary director of research at the RAFT (Restoration of Appearance and Function Trust) Institute for Plastic Surgery at Mount Vernon Hospital, Northwood, London, where he produced a low air-loss mattress to prevent pressure sores, based on the reverse principle of the hovercraft.

See Hampson (2004); www.raft.
ac.uk/common/jts.html (visited
1 August 2006). See also Kenedi
et al. (eds) (1976) and Figure 20.

Sir Herbert Seddon
Kt CMG DM FRCS (1903–77)
was Resident Surgeon at the
country branch [Stanmore,
Middlesex] of the RNOH from
1931 to 1939 and Nuffield
Professor of Orthopaedic Surgery,
University of Oxford, from 1940
to 1948. He was appointed
Director of Studies at the Institute
of Orthopaedics, University of
London, a joint appointment
between the RNOH and the
Institute, from 1948 to 1965 and
was Professor of Orthopaedics there
from 1965 until his retirement
in 1967. He was a member of
the Medical Research Council,
from 1956–59 and was interested
in African and tropical medical
problems. See Seddon and Scales
(1949); Seddon (1950); Nicholson
and Seddon (1957); Parsons and
Seddon (1968).

Mr Edgar William Somerville
MB FRCSEd (1913–96) qualified
in 1938, and served in the Royal
Air Force until he was demobilized
in 1946. He was Consultant
Surgeon at the Wingfield Morris
Hospital, Oxford (renamed the
Nuffield Orthopaedic Centre in
1956), Oxford, until his retirement

in 1977, specializing in the
treatment of children's deformities
and the pathology and treatment
of congenital dislocation of the
hip. He was Editorial Secretary
and then Vice-President of the
BOA; President of the Orthopaedic
Section of the Royal Society of
Medicine, the British Orthopaedic
Research Society and the ABC
Orthopaedic Club. See Girdlestone
and Somerville (1952) and
Somerville (1982).

Mr Ian B M Stephen
MB FRCS (b. 1944) trained at
Cambridge, Bristol, Exeter and
Montreal, Canada, was Consultant
in Orthopaedic and Trauma
Surgery, East Kent Hospitals,
from 1983 to 2002 and Clinical
Director, Trauma and Orthopaedic
Surgery, 2000 to 2002, and has
been an independent consultant
orthopaedic foot and ankle
surgeon, Margate, Kent, since
2002. He is Past President of the
Orthopaedic Section, Royal Society
of Medicine, Archivist of the BOA,
and member of the Expert Witness
Institute.

Mr Malcolm Swann
FRCS (b. 1931) was Consultant
Orthopaedic Surgeon to the
Windsor Group of Hospitals from
1967 until his retirement in 2001.
His special interest is in paediatric
orthopaedics and he worked closely

with Professor Barbara Ansell, the Paediatric Rheumatologist, and later established a surgical service for patients with juvenile chronic arthritis at the Canadian Red Cross Hospital at Taplow. See Ansell *et al.* (1997).

Professor Alan Swanson
PhD DSc FREng FIMechE (b. 1931) graduated in mechanical engineering from Imperial College, London, in 1952. He worked in engineering laboratories at Bristol Aircraft (1955–58), was appointed Lecturer in Mechanical Engineering, Imperial College, in 1958, Reader in Biomechanics, 1969 and Professor of Biomechanics from 1974 until his retirement in 1997. With Michael Freeman he founded the Biomechanics Unit at Imperial College in 1964, where work was done on the mechanical properties of bone and articular cartilage, internal fixation devices and joint replacements.

Sir Rodney Sweetnam
KCVO CBE FRCS FRCSEd (b. 1927) was Consultant Orthopaedic Surgeon to the Middlesex Hospital and University College Hospital, London, from 1974 to 1992, later Emeritus. He served as Consultant Adviser in Orthopaedic Surgery to the Department of Health (1981–90);

Orthopaedic Surgeon to the Queen (1983–92); President of the BOA (1985); President of the Royal College of Surgeons of England (1995–98) and a Fellow of UCL. See Wiles and Sweetnam (1965); and Hughes and Sweetnam (eds) (1980).

Mr Keith Tucker
MB FRCS (b. 1945) was Senior House Officer to Ken McKee in 1970; Senior Registrar at St Bartholomew's Hospital, London, Surgical Training Programme in Orthopaedics, including Senior Registrarships to Messrs Lettin, Read, Phillips, Watson-Farrar, Taylor, Wilson and Kemp, from 1973 to 1977. He has been Consultant Orthopaedic Surgeon, Norfolk and Norwich University Hospital, Norwich, since 1978. He is a founder member of the British Hip Society and has been Honorary Secretary (1998–2005) and Vice President (2005–07) and will serve as President in 2007/08; elected a member of the Steering Committee of the National Joint Registry in 2006; Chairman of the Orthopaedic Data Evaluation Panel (ODEP) since 2002; and BOA representative to the MDA/MHRA since 1994.

Sir Reginald Watson-Jones

Kt FRCS HonFRCSEd
(1902–72) qualified and trained
at Liverpool University, and
later held lectureships and
demonstratorships in anatomy,
physiology and physiotherapy
there. He was resident house
surgeon at the RNOH and clinical
assistant at Great Ormond Street
Hospital for Children, returning to
Liverpool in 1926 as senior surgical
tutor and registrar at the Royal
Infirmary, where he was later an
orthopaedic surgeon. He organized
the Royal Air Force's orthopaedic
services during the war; was Hon.
Consultant, later Director, of
the Orthopaedic and Accident
Department, London Hospital,
from 1943; orthopaedic surgeon to
King George VI, 1946 to 1952 and
to the Queen from 1952. He was
the first British Editor, *Journal of
Bone and Joint Surgery,* from 1947;
President, BOA, 1952–53; Senior
Vice-President, Royal College of
Surgeons of England, 1953–54;
Member of the Court of Examiners
of the RCS, and Hunterian
Orator, 1959; and President of the
Orthopaedic Section of the Royal
Society of Medicine, 1956.

Mr Victor H Wheble

FRCSEd (b. 1919) qualified at
Oxford and trained at King's
College Hospital Medical School,
London, and served as a member
of the Baptist Missionary Society
in the Belgian Congo. Following
a serious illness in Africa, he was
Registrar and Senior Registrar at
Manfield Orthopaedic Hospital,
Northampton. He was appointed
Consultant Orthopaedic Surgeon
at Ashton-under-Lyne General
Hospital, near Manchester, from
1960 to 1984. He was a Visiting
Fellow and Lecturer at the
University of Salford, undertook
research at UMIST with Dr Jan
Skorecki, and had close ties with
Professor Garth Hastings at the
Biomedical Engineering Unit,
Staffordshire Polytechnic, Stoke-
on-Trent [now Staffordshire
University]. He has been a member,
and frequently Chairman, of
many national and international
committees concerned with the
standardization of surgical implants
from 1972 to 2001, representing
the BOA and subsequently the
Royal College of Surgeons of
England. See Wheble (1994).

Mr Philip Wiles

FRCS (1899–1967) served in the
Army and the Royal Flying Corps,
joined his father in the City of
London, and came to medicine late,
a mature student at the Middlesex
Hospital, London. He became a
Consultant there at age 36. He
served in the Middle East and
India in the Second World War,
becoming a brigadier. Retiring early,

he moved to Jamaica, becoming Chairman of the Scientific Research Council and encouraged the growth of the medical school. His textbook on orthopaedics ran to four editions and several reprintings. He was the treasurer to the British edition of the *Journal of Bone and Joint Surgery,* became President of the BOA. See Seddon (1967).

Mr James Noel (Ginger) Wilson
OBE ChM FRCS (1919–2006) co-designer with John Scales of the Stanmore Hip System, qualified at Birmingham, joining the Royal Army Medical Corps in 1943, with the 1st Airborne Division in Europe and Norway. He was Orthopaedic Registrar at Robert Jones and Agnes Hunt Orthopaedic Hospital, Oswestry, 1949–52, then Consultant at Cardiff Royal Infirmary, and BOA Travelling Fellow to the USA in 1954. He was Consultant Orthopaedic Surgeon and a Director of the Accident Service at the RNOH, London, and Stanmore, from 1955–84, and Assistant Director of Postgraduate Training at RNOH from 1968–72, Clinical Teacher at the Institute of Orthopaedics, University of London and Consultant Orthopaedic Surgeon to the National Hospital for Nervous Diseases, Queen Square, London, from 1962–84. He worked extensively in the Third World developing orthopaedic training programmes, even after retirement, and served as Professor of Orthopaedics at Addis Ababa University, Ethiopia in 1989. He was a founding member of World Orthopaedic Concern (WOC) and edited the *WOC Newsletter* for over a decade in his retirement; President of the Orthopaedic Section of the Royal Society of Medicine, later Honorary member; Editorial Secretary of the BOA (1974–78), and Vice-Chairman of the IMPACT Foundation (1985–2001). See Watson-Jones (1976, 1982); Owen (2006).

Mr Michael Wilson
MA (Glasgow) (b. 1956), 'Ginger' Wilson's son.

Professor B Michael Wroblewski
FRCSEd (b. 1934) trained at Leeds Medical School and after posts at Leeds, Manchester, Oswestry, Wrightington and Birmingham, he was appointed Consultant Orthopaedic Surgeon at the Centre for Hip Surgery, Wrightington Hospital, Lancashire, from 1973 to 2004. He was also External Professor of Orthopaedic Biomechanics at the University of Leeds in 1992. He helped to establish the John Charnley Research Institute and Charitable Trust in 1992, which has funded 25 Clinical Research Fellows, 1987–2001. See Wroblewski (1990, 2002).

Glossary*

arthrodesis of the hip
The surgical fusion of the femur (thigh bone) to the pelvis, in which the hip joint surfaces are surgically removed and the denuded joint surfaces pressed together and fixed with special plates and screws. Also known as fusion.

arthroplasty
Surgical replacement of all or part of the hip joint with an artificial device to decrease the friction and wear between the femoral head prosthesis and the cartilage of the acetabulum or its prosthetic lining. Metal, polyethylene and ceramic or combinations have been used.

bone cement, self-hardening
A cement which hardens when its components are mixed together. No external physical agency, such as heat or UV light, is needed to initiate the hardening process. In implant surgery, the hardening process is usually one of polymerization.

Birmingham resurfacing arthroplasty (BSA)
A metal-on-metal prosthesis, introduced in 1991 by Derek McMinn, Birmingham Nuffield Hospital, and manufactured by Midland Medical Technologies Ltd, which covers the hip joint surfaces with accurately machined, large-headed metal prostheses, instead of replacing them. The acetabular component is fixed with a **hydroxyapatite coating,** while the femoral component is cemented in place. See McMinn *et al.* (1996); Appendix 3, page 106.

British Hip Society
Michael Freeman, Robin Ling and Hugh Phillips founded the Hip Society in 1989, an affiliate of the BOA. Phillips was involved in the inception of the National Joint Register, the Capital hip enquiry, and wrote the first edition of *The Guide to Best Practice in Hip Surgery*, published by the BHS in 1999.

CE marking or EC mark
The letters CE are the abbreviation of French phrase Conformité Européene or European Conformity. Initially the term was 'EC Mark', replaced by 'CE Marking' in 1993 by European Directive 93/68/EEC. A product with this mark has a manufacturer's declaration that the product complies with the

*Terms in bold appear in the Glossary as separate entries

essential requirements of the relevant European health, safety and environmental protection legislation, and conforms to European product directives. For further details see www.dti. gov.uk/innovation/strd/cemark/ page11646.html (visited 11 September 2006).

cobalt–chromium (Co–Cr) alloys

A family of alloys with cobalt as the main constituent, used in general engineering for resistance to wear and corrosion, and in dentistry and orthopaedics.

corrosion

A reaction between the surface of a metal or alloy and the surrounding medium (air, liquid or both). The resulting metallic oxides, chlorides etc., may remain firmly attached or may readily detach, which makes the alloy unsuitable for implants, whereas the former characteristic makes certain alloys ideal for use as implants.

endosteal surface of the femur

The inner surface of the bone around the marrow cavity.

Exeter hip

The original, made in EN58J steel [BS 970 Grade 316S16, austenitic, non-magnetic, offers high resistance to corrosion] was available for use in clinical practice from autumn 1970, manufactured by the London

Splint Company (now Howmedica UK Ltd) in polished stainless steel with a head size of 29.75mm, cemented with acrylic bone cement and in two sizes (standard and lightweight). The cup was made from high-density polyethylene in three sizes. See Ling (1997): 7, 10–11. See also www.exeterhip. co.uk/ex_pag_redirect-about-us.htm (visited 29 June 2006) and Figure 21.

Fluorosint®

A proprietary plastic mixture where synthetically-manufactured mica is chemically linked to **polytetrafluoroethylene (PTFE),** resulting in properties not normally attainable in reinforced PTFE.

Girdlestone

A resection **arthroplasty** of the hip, where the resected part of the ball or head of the thigh bone (femur) and the rest of the femur is left loose, allowing some movement between the femur and hip (acetabulum). The muscle and soft tissues, including the scar of the previous operations, infection or inflammation prevent the femur riding up a great deal past the hip bone socket. The leg shortening can be several inches. The movement of the pseudoarthrosis allows the patient to sit more easily in a chair than with a fused hip. See the classic article by Professor Gathorne

Robert Girdlestone (1881–1950), the first Nuffield Professor of Orthopaedic surgery at the University of Oxford, who devised this treatment for tuberculosis of the hip and later has been used in severe osteoarthritis and more recently as a last resort for failed total hip replacements that could not be revised. Girdlestone (1943).

hemi-arthroplasty

Surgical replacement of only the head of the femur. It is often called an Austin-Moore or Thompson. A bipolar hemi-arthroplasty uses a femoral prosthesis with an articulating acetabular part, but not fixed to the acetabulum.

high-density polyethylene (HDP)
See **ultra-high molecular weight polyethylene (UHMWPE)**

hydroxyapatite coating (HAC)

A bioactive material applied to uncemented prosthesis to encourage the bonding of the bone to secure the implant.

International Organization for Standardization (ISO)

An international non-governmental organization that began as the International Electrotechnical Commission (IEC) in 1906 (later the International Federation of the National Standardizing Associations (ISA), 1926–42). A new postwar organization, the ISO, started in 1947 to coordinate and unify industrial standards. The abbreviation ISO is based on the Greek *isos*, meaning 'equal'.

Journal of Bone and Joint Surgery (JBJS)

Originated as the *Transactions of the American Orthopedic Association* and vol. 1 contained the proceedings of the meetings of 1887 and 1888. Volume 16 (1903) of the *Transactions* is also vol. 1 of the *American Journal of Orthopedic Surgery*. It became the official publication of the British Orthopaedic Association in 1919 and the name changed to the *Journal of Orthopaedic Surgery*, vol. 1 (new series), with the present title the *Journal of Bone and Joint Surgery* adopted in 1922. In 1948, the A (American) and B (British) volumes were established, while the American Orthopedic Association remained the owner until an independent non-profit corporation was created.

Küntscher nail, or intramedullary rod

A hollow rod of varying lengths and diameters secured to the medulla, the hollow cavity inside the femur, which was in frequent use until the 1970s. Named after Gerhard Küntscher, a German surgeon who used it. Some attribute its use to explain why German soldiers in the

Second World War were back in action a few months after fractured femurs, whereas the Allied soldiers were back, in traction.

laminar ultraclean air flow systems

Unidirectional clean-air systems for surgical theatres that became widely used in the 1960s, designed for 300+ air changes per hour, re-circulating the air through filters and flowing horizontally through a wall module or downwards from an air inlet overhead. These systems led to very low numbers of airborne bacteria. See Lowbury and Lidwell (1978); see also note 158.

low-frictional arthroplasty

Sir John Charnley's operation for **total hip replacement,** available from 1962, cemented using finger packing. See Charnley (1979).

medialized cups

Acetabular prosthesis inserted deeply.

morselized graft

A cancellaus bone graft impacted into the proximal femur. The bone is usually taken from the femoral head in a primary replacement, and the proximal femur, if it is a revision. The bone is chopped into chips using a bone mill and used as a graft. A cadaver graft is used if an allograft is not available.

Ortron

A **cobalt–chromium alloy** originally developed by Krupp in Germany for dental implants and has excellent corrosion resistance. Adopted by DePuy for use in the Charnley prosthesis after 1990.

osteolysis

The dissolution of bone through disease, commonly due to infection or by loss of blood supply to the bone, and a common cause of loosening; a major failure in **total hip replacement.**

polyethylene

A polymer of ethylene (C_2H_4) widely used for buckets. Higher levels of polymerization allow closer packing of the molecules with fewer voids, and the resulting high- or **ultra-high molecular weight polyethylene** has improved wear resistance.

polymethylmethacrylate cement

Made by mixing a powder polymethylmethacrylate plus an activator with a fluid methylmethacrylate plus an inhibitor in a bowl with a spoon and spatula. The mixture becomes creamy and then doughy. After three to four minutes it begins to set and as it does so, it becomes hot, producing a characteristic smell. The material, having become viscous, is plastic, then elastic, before becoming solid.

polytetrafluoroethylene (PTFE)

A thermoplastic discovered unexpectedly in 1938 when a cylinder stored under pressure was cut open. It became available commercially in the US and the UK in 1948. It is resistant to high and low temperatures, has low loss dielectric properties over a wide frequency range, a chemical inertness and anti-stick properties, which led to its early use in the aerospace industry and as non-stick cookware (Teflon® pans were first sold at Christmas 1961) and plumber's thread tape. See www.plastiquarian.com/ptfe.htm (visited 20 June 2006).

proximal stress shielding

This occurs when the stiff proximal end of a femoral prosthesis transmits most of the load between the hip joint and the femoral shaft, and the surrounding bone, being subjected to abnormally low stresses, is resorbed over time by the normal remodelling process, which responds to stress levels, among other things.

RNOH

see **Royal National Orthopaedic Hospital**

radiolucent/radio-opaque

A radiolucent zone in an X-ray permits the passage of X-rays, unlike one that is radio-opaque.

rasp or broach

An instrument used for clearing the femoral canal.

reamer

A burr-like instrument used during the hip replacement operation to remove arthritic bone from the acetabulum, by rasping; or to shape the medullary canal. An acetabular reamer is hemispherical; the femoral is straight, tapered or pin-shaped. See Figure 22.

Royal National Orthopaedic Hospital (RNOH), Stanmore

RNOH was recognized by the University of London in 1946 as a postgraduate teaching hospital and the Institute of Orthopaedics and Musculoskeletal Science (IOMS) was founded there, initially located in Great Portland Street, London. By 1948 most of the facilities had moved to Stanmore, Middlesex, called the country branch of the hospital. A unit looking into research on plastics began in 1948, renamed Biomechanics and Surgical Materials in 1954, later Biomedical Engineering, and led by Professor John Scales bringing together the various applications of engineering to orthopaedic problems. Stanmore Implants Worldwide (SIW) was formed for the manufacture of specialized prosthetic implants, which became a limited company in 1996. A collection of radiographs has been held in the Wellcome Museum of Orthopaedics and the Radiological Department for the Museum of Orthopaedic Radiology, supported by £5300 of grants from the Wellcome Trust to adapt and equip rooms at Great Portland Street, and opened by Sir Henry Dale in 1956. See Cholmeley (1982).

self-curing acrylic bone cement
see **polymethylmethacrylate cement**

Shenton's line
A radiographic, curved line formed by the top of the obturator foramen and the inner side of the neck of the femur, used to determine the relationship of the head of the femur to the acetabulum. Also known as the Ménard-Shenton-Makkas line, after Edward Warren Hine Shenton. See Renner (1925).

slit sampler
An instrument which sucks air through a narrow slit onto the surface of a culture medium, rotated slowly, just below the slit. See Bourdillon *et al.* (1941) and Figure 25.

Staphylococcus epidermidis
A gram-positive pathogenic bacterium common in medical device-associated infections. *S. epidermidis* normally lives on the skin and only causes infection if introduced around a foreign body, such as an implant. See www.ebi. ac.uk/2can/genomes/genomes. html?http://www.ebi.ac.uk/2can/ genomes/bacteria/Staphylococcus_ epidermidis.html (visited 1 August 2006).

Stanmore
see **Royal National Orthopaedic Hospital**

Stanmore hip
The original Stanmore prosthesis was available from spring 1963. See Figure 17 and Appendix 3, page 104.

survivorship analysis
A statistical method that looks at the frequency of revision of a prosthesis by the number of years of clinical implantation, taking into consideration the loss of patients at follow-up due to death and other factors.

Teflon®
The trade name for a family of **PTFE** resins produced by DuPont, Wilmington, Delaware, USA.

Thackray's
Charles F Thackray Ltd of Leeds started as retail pharmacists in 1862, diversifying into surgical equipment and orthopaedics in 1947. They manufactured the Charnley prosthesis from 1963 until 1990 when Thackray's was acquired by DePuy, the US subsidiary of a

private German firm, Boehringer Mannheim, in 1990, taken over by Johnson & Johnson. The Charnley total hip replacement is currently manufactured under the name of DePuy International. See www.jnjgateway.com/home.jhtml?loc=G BENG&page=viewContent&cont entId=09008b9880bba4bc (visited 19 October 2006). The Thackray Museum, Leeds, was established in a former workhouse building of the St James's Hospital, Leeds, by Paul Thackray, a former director and major shareholder in Thackray's in 1997, initially as an archive of the company.

titanium (Ti)
A light metal with high resistance to corrosion. Since the Kroll process was developed in 1937, it can be made in considerable quantities, mostly used by the aircraft industry, the chemical industry and for medical applications.

total hip replacement
The surgical replacement of the head of the femur and the acetabulum with manufactured components.

tribology
The study of mechanisms of friction, lubrication and wear of interacting surfaces that are in relative motion. See Dowson (ed.) (1998).

trochanteric osteotomy
An operation to cut the greater trochanter, with all its muscles attached, from the femur to expose the hip joint, or to alter its mechanics. See Wroblewski (1990): 19–28.

ultra-high molecular weight polyethylene (UHMWPE)
A polymer used in orthopaedics that is classified as a linear homopolymer formed from ethylene (C_2H_4). The densely packed and curled molecular chains give it good wear characteristics. Irradiation for sterilization should be in a vacuum, otherwise the chains of the molecules unravel. It has been used in hip replacement since 1961 when Charnley used it for its low-friction and high-wear resistance properties for his metal-on-plastic hip joint. Since then it has been used in a large range of joint replacements for the hip, knee, ankle, elbow and shoulder.

Vitallium®
A trademarked alloy of 60 per cent cobalt, 20 per cent chromium, and 5 per cent molybdenum used for prostheses, implants and instruments since 1936. See Venable and Stuck (1943).

Index: Subject

Index: Names

Biographical notes appear in bold

Key to cover photographs

Front cover, top to bottom

Mr Alan Lettin (Chair)

Mr Peter Ring

Mrs Phyllis Hampson

Mr Victor Wheble

Back cover, top to bottom

Sir Rodney Sweetnam

Lady Charnley, Mr Reg Elson, Mr Tristram Charnley

Professor Michael Freeman

Professor Alan Swanson

Lightning Source UK Ltd.
Milton Keynes UK
30 October 2009

145609UK00001B/84/A